BORN ON THE WRONG PLANET

"A crisp, funny book by a bright, successful young woman, Erika Hammerschmidt's *Born on the Wrong Planet* is a must-read for parents, therapists, educators, and the afflicted!"

— *Linda Y. Callaghan, MD*

"Erika Hammerschmidt is able to convey the challenges that she and others truly face on a daily level. *Born on the Wrong Planet* reaffirms understanding of her and others' struggles, and reveals the thinking and feeling process as a very genuine one that is easily misperceived by others."

— *Don Taylor, MSW*

"Erika Hammerschmidt's style allowed me to feel as though I were walking in her shoes, experiencing her pain. *Born on the Wrong Planet* can definitely help others living with similar situations, their caregivers, and those who simply want to understand for their own life enrichment."

— *Gail Korza, MA, MHRS*

TO MELISSA
GOOD LUCK!

Born on the Wrong Planet

Second Edition

Erika Hammerschmidt

TYBORNE HILL PUBLISHERS

PALO ALTO, CALIFORNIA

Tyborne Hill Publishers
2730 South Court Street
Palo Alto, California 94306
Visit our website at www.tybornehill.com

Editor: *Audrey DeLaMartre*
Production Editor and Internal Design: *Carolyn Serebreny*
Cover Design: *Sonia Kruglova*

Definitions of Asperger's Syndrome used in the Appendix from the online Asperger Syndrome Information and Support website, http://www.udel.edu/bkirby/asperger. Used with permission. Definition of Tourette's Syndrome in the Appendix from the online website of the Tourette's Syndrome Association, Inc., http://www.tsa-usa.org. Used with permission. Definitions of the diagnostic features of Asperger's Disorder and Tourette's Disorder, Obsessive-Compulsive Disorder, and Attention-Deficit/Hyperactivity Disorder from the *Diagnostic and Statistical Manual of Mental Disorders* of the American Psychiatric Association. Used with permission.

ISBN: 0-9748570-6-8

Printed in the United States of America

To Mom and Dad, for helping me through the toughest times.
To Karl, for making sure I don't take myself too seriously.
To Martha, Steve, Matthew, Sonja, Peter, Elsie, Tosh,
Puff, and Sparky, for being my second family.
To my friends, for showing me I'm not alone.

Foreword

In terms of social rules, humans have some of the most complicated codes on our planet. Other species have social codes, it's true, such as how close and from which side another animal may approach; what constitutes aggression; what constitutes acceptable mating behavior; and, in general, what behaviors are not acceptable. While these codes can be extremely complicated, usually lower-order animals direct their social behaviors toward survival, and the penalties for violating them are immediate and often lethal. Few lower-order animals survive for long who don't grasp simple social codes.

Human behavior is different. We have developed extremely convoluted and often obscure social codes. For example, what we say, how we dress, wear adornments, and paint our bodies have connected to survival behaviors—a hazardous connection. We restrict who may wear what, who must cover what, and who may say what. To make it worse, our norms vary from one human culture to another, and change with the day.

Over the centuries we have developed sets of social interaction rules so complex that they take years and experience to learn. Unfortunately, mastering them defines the individual in human society, regardless of the individual's other qualities. Without mastery of our created social norms, individuals are not allowed to participate in society fully, even if we perceive that they have something to offer.

We teach our children to choose words that don't offend and behavior that "respects other's boundaries," even when the words that give offense change on a regular basis, and boundaries are a nebulous and culture-dependent concept that differs in other countries and social contexts.

Ordinarily we don't kill people who violate our social norms, although in some extreme cases we do; however, we have countless unspoken penalties for crossing society's boundaries, which we expect children to learn by age six. Woe be unto the child who has not.

Unfortunately, as a society we make a fatal—actually primitive— assumption that every child can learn our codes with ease. That is not true.

Some children (especially children with disorders that manifest in early childhood, like Asperger's Syndrome, Tourette's Syndrome, Attention Deficit Disorder (ADD), Attention Deficit/Hyperactivity Disorder (ADHD), Obsessive-Compulsive Disorder (OCD), and so on, as defined in the *Diagnostic and Statistical Manual of Mental Disorders* of the American Psychiatric Association) are hard-put to understand the social processes, much less conform to them readily.

What is our enlightened response to people who cannot learn our social guidelines? In my darkest moments I think lower-order animals might have a kinder solution than do we humans. Instead of killing children who can't learn our complex guidelines by age six or sooner, we *torture* them, often for a lifetime. Our social instrument of torture, cruelest of any, is ridicule by other children—the peer group, progressing from there to more sophisticated patterns of oppression!

So-called normal children discern early the differences between themselves and children afflicted with any kind of disorder, emotional or physical, and persecute, ridicule, and taunt them with practical jokes and sometimes worse.

Sadly, schools, geared normally to a narrow range of acceptable behavior, have little tolerance for anything outside of that conventional range. Hence, unconventional individuals are referred to special education classes, which don't necessarily separate the mentally challenged from those otherwise afflicted, and where often there is no real understanding (beyond knowledge of the symptoms) of the afflictions, or that an individual so afflicted can be a successful, productive, and worthwhile person.

Erika Hammerschmidt, laden with the unwieldy combination of such disorders and a superior intellect, felt she was living in an alien society. The fact that she has intelligence within the genius range made it more unbearable, because no matter what those so afflicted do to be accepted, they meet only more ridicule.

It is easy to love children with pleasing personalities who don't challenge our patience. We don't, usually, extend this easy love or acceptance to those unfortunate enough to be born with conditions that provoke aversion, laughter, or embarrassment. Exclusion is a thoughtless form of abuse that is easy to fall into.

Sadly, these afflicted children don't understand other's cruelty and rejection. Generally they feel the cruelty is their fault, internalize the feeling as inadequacy and shame, and learn defense mechanisms such as repression, dissociation, and magical thinking.

Erika Hammerschmidt, however, got lucky! Many parents and teachers are preoccupied with loving and controlling children and their situations, and are not alert to obvious signs that a child's behaviors can alienate that child from peers. However, Hammerschmidt's parents and a few of her teachers realized the need to feel normal and loved, not naughty or a troublesome burden. With this recognition, Hammerschmidt escaped the depression, anxiety, and acting out that creates more alienation and rejection.

Erika Hammerschmidt has forged new links and opened doors by writing her story. If we are alert enough to benefit from her courage this world can be a better place for all of us.

LINDA Y. CALLAGHAN, M.D.

Dr. Callaghan is a psychiatrist in private practice in Traverse City, Michigan, and the author of *Inrage: Healing the Hidden Rage of Child Sexual Abuse* (Tyborne Hill Publishers, 2003).

Introduction

I wanted to go to my high school prom dressed in a homemade alien costume, but my family talked me out of it. They said it would ruin the experience for other people. After much protest, I gave in, acknowledging my lesser authority on the psychology of humans. I went in a beautiful red gown that cost my grandmother hundreds of dollars and had such a tight bodice that I started feeling sick during the festivities.

To be completely honest, I am not sure that I wouldn't have gotten sick in the alien costume, too. But the college Halloween dance of 1999, to which I did wear the alien costume, turned out to be the first school dance I have ever truly enjoyed. In fact, every time I've worn that costume since then, I have had fun.

I can only assume that the fun comes from being dressed the right way for once in my life; from saying to the world openly that I don't belong in the body I was born in, and I don't know what my real body is like, but here's a guess—this costume is closer than anything else I've found. I'm not quite ready for species-transplant surgery, but I'm sure I would fit better somewhere else. Planet Earth does not always feel like home to souls who are labeled Asperger's Syndrome, Tourette's Syndrome, OCD, ADD, ADHD, or All of the Above.[1]

---

[1] Diagnostic terms in this book are defined in the Appendix on page 115.

Those of us with a small helping of everything have a particularly hard time. Our actions can be close enough to the norm that we look like misbehaving normal people, but we don't quite fit in with ordinary society, or with more severely afflicted people. And the variety of our disorders causes the same dilemma as having a multi-racial background. With which part do we identify? Too often, we end up in the miscellaneous category.

We all have places we can belong, if we create them. In these pages, you'll find my views of Earth from everywhere I've been. This is my story of feeling that I belonged in another world, of taking refuge in worlds I built for myself, and finally, of learning to live in the world where I was born!

Erika Hammerschmidt
April 2005

A Problem Child

Living in a household where an expression of feeling could start temper tantrums, Mary had learned not to show her own emotions. She did not sigh or groan. Her chest constricted and she let out a long breath, leaving an aching vacuum behind her breastbone that refilled only gradually as she read the letter.

"Another one?" said her husband, looking at her anxiously.

Mary nodded and passed the letter to him. He read it, and then did sigh.

"Another one. And they're actually asking us to come this time. It must be serious."

"I'll go," said Mary, pushing aside clutter to make a place for the letter on the bedside table.

The kindergarten was in a small building, and the children stayed mainly in one big room with several sections: a play kitchen, a block-building area, a book corner, a shelf full of math toys. Mary gave the faintest smile of approval, seeing the tiny one-centimeter cubes that taught about the metric system; the colorful pie-shaped transparencies representing fractions; the little tabs of paper that were black on one side and red on the other.

Mary left her daughter with the other children. Like a drop of oil in a cup of water, the girl meandered slightly apart from them, floating in her own bubble of space.

Mary approached a teacher who was setting out black and red tabs on the math table. "I heard things aren't going as well as they could?" she asked, feigning lightness.

"Honestly, I don't know what's going on with that kid," said the teacher, brushing permed hair out of her eyes. "She can't follow any instructions at all. The simplest things, even. She talks back, she won't pay any attention ... I'm afraid this is really a problem child."

Mary stifled a sigh in the way that had become almost natural to her.

"The last straw was yesterday. It was nap time, and I said, 'Now lay down, all of you.' And she looks up at me and says, in this really defiant, rude voice, 'You're wrong! You should have said *lie* down.'"

A spark of amusement got to Mary's eyes before she could stop it, and the teacher scowled. "It was really impertinent, it really was. I mean, she's five! Younger than the other kids, even! And she thinks she has any business talking back to teachers!"

"Is anything else the matter?"

"Everything! She won't play with the others. When she does, she hits them. She bites, too. She talks back all the time. She just ignores everything when we have a lesson. She won't use the bathrooms. You must have noticed that she's practically jumping around with crossed legs by the time you come to pick her up in the evening."

"What color are the toilets?"

"What color? Perfectly regular color, white with black seats."

"Not beige?"

"No. Why?"

"She won't use beige toilets."

"Huh! Well, they aren't. They're perfectly fine, even built extra small for kindergartners. I can't see why she would have a problem with them. But she does. She has a problem with everything! She makes everything so much harder than it has to be. Just stay here a day, and you'll see."

Nap time. Snack time. Play time. Things seemed very organized in kindergarten. Mary sat in a corner, watching the children play. Here, a girl put a doll to bed; there, some boys built a castle of blocks.

It all seemed very normal, Mary's eyes turned to her own daughter. The five-year-old was wandering among the different play areas, never stopping, never seeming particularly interested in one or another of the activities offered. Quietly she was talking to herself, a real monologue with pauses and exaggerated facial expressions and changes in voice tone, as if she were telling a story to a still younger child.

There must be some place, Mary thought. There must be some place for a five-year-old girl who makes up stories in her head and knows the difference between transitive and intransitive verbs better than her teachers do! Some school where she can fit in.

"Math time." The children were herded to the big kidney-shaped table by the blackboard, where ten little tabs of paper, black on one side, red on the other, were set out at each student's place.

"You know the rules," the teacher began. "We'll have math time for 30 minutes. Today we're still learning about adding. We're using these today." She held up a handful of the paper tabs.

Mary narrowed her eyes just slightly, an expression of emotion that no one saw.

"Now you have a minute to do the first problem. Set out three tabs with the red side up, and then set out two next to them, with the black side up."

Each child obeyed, except the five-year-old near the end of the table. Sucking the thumb of one hand, absently arranging the bits of paper in various patterns, she kept whispering to herself out of the corners of her mouth, completely detached.

"Has everybody got them set out the way I said? Everybody? How about you?" The teacher paused, leaning over Mary's daughter.

The little girl looked up, barely pulling her thumb out of her mouth. "What?" she murmured.

"Do you have the papers set out the right way?"

"What way?"

"No, I can see you don't. Well, I'll come back to you." The teacher let out a heavy sigh and went on to another student.

After a moment, apparently satisfied that all the children who mattered had done the experiment correctly, she announced, "All right! Now, how many pieces of paper do you have out, in all?"

A moment of silence, and then, a murmuring voice interrupted its own soliloquy and said, "Ten."

"Ten? How did you get ten?"

"I counted them. One, two, three, four, five, six, seven, eight, nine, ten."

An even heavier sigh. "You counted all the ones we gave you. I meant, count the ones that you set out in the way I told you."

"But I didn't."

"I can see that." Having exhausted her sighing vocabulary, the teacher simply rolled her eyes. "Does anyone else have an answer?"

"Five," volunteered one child.

"Great work! Can the rest of you see how we got that number?" She spread her nail-polished fingers out around the paper tabs of the child who had answered correctly. "Let's count them, okay? One ... two ... three ... four ... five."

Mary fidgeted. Her daughter was folding her tiny squares of paper on the diagonal, and holding them between her thumbs and forefingers, squeezing so that they opened and closed like little pointed mouths. One in each hand, they appeared to carry on a conversation with each other.

"Now, let's set out three with the black side up, and two with the red side ... *Stop that!* These are for math, they are not toys!" The teacher turned on Mary's daughter, who made a face and set the pieces of paper down, hesitantly, defiantly. "Stop playing around, and stop sucking your thumb, and be quiet and do the work! Set down three black and two red, now!"

The girl sullenly started counting out paper squares, and the lesson went on.

For half an hour they repeated the same exercise, only the numbers varied — three black and two red, four black and one red, four red and one black, two black and one red, two red and one black, two black and two red, one black and one red, on and on and on.

Mary saw her daughter disobey, or misunderstand, a dozen times. She made a pile of two red and a pile of three black, when the pieces were clearly meant to be set out next to each other. She replied that there were two red and three black, instead of saying that there were five. She chewed on one of the pieces. She ignored several rounds of the exercise completely, staring into space, murmuring around her thumb.

Mary didn't blame her!

"Math time is over! Now it's bathroom time," announced the teacher. "Line up, everybody, and we'll all walk down to the bathroom."

Mary followed the tide of moving children until she reached the teacher's side. Her little girl gravitated toward her and clung, one drop of oil finding another in an ocean of water.

"Excuse me," Mary said, emotionlessness and friendliness still precariously balanced. "I think I'll just take her home now, if you don't mind. I think I've seen enough to understand what you're talking about."

"Oh, good," said the teacher, smiling tightly. "I hope you have a long talk with her. Good night."

In the car, driving home with her daughter, Mary finally let her feelings out. Only in words, granted; she kept her voice tone close to neutral, even cheerful. But she said the things she had been wanting to say.

"Regimentation ... kindergarten children's attention spans ... thirty minutes of math! I don't think I could stand to watch that again. It hurt. All those fun, entertaining, really amazingly helpful little math toys, and then they use them like that. It hurt. It could have been made fun for them—all those children who are learning that math is 30 minutes of 'Now two red and two black. Now one red and three black'—"

"And their toilets are the wrong size," put in her daughter.

"Yes! And their toilets are the wrong size. Too small. Like their minds." Mary managed a laugh. "They think you're a problem child. They think every problem child has to be treated exactly the same way: yell at her, send a note home, make the parents have a long talk with her. Well, this is my long talk: You're not just some problem child. You're not some teacher's cookie-cutter model of a bad kid. You're you. Don't worry, I'll find the right school for you, if I have to look all over the city."

Mary pulled into a gas station and led her daughter inside to the bathroom.

Parents

Before I was born, Mom and Dad sometimes were asked, "Do you want it to be a girl or a boy?" They said, "It doesn't matter, as long as we can tell which it is."

They thought that was clever, and they got their wish: at my birth, they were quite able to identify me as a girl. But then they spent my childhood making sure no one else could make the same identification.

Not that they dressed me as a boy; the clothes and hairstyle they chose for me were deliberately gender-neutral. They were afraid of child molesters. A child molester, they said, is usually interested in either males or females, and will leave you alone if there's uncertainty.

And it worked. I never once got sexually molested by an adult. Just emotionally molested by other children, *nonstop* through grade school. It's amazing how important genders are to people who haven't even gotten to puberty yet. They couldn't stop teasing me, and I couldn't stop being hurt by it. By the time I realized the entertainment potential of being able to pass for male, I was already starting to look too female for it to work.

I can think of many such examples of my parents' eccentric but very real concern for my wellbeing; not only protectiveness, but a deep need for my happiness. Sometimes their attempts to make me happy only annoyed me, but always they had my best interests in mind, and often I was grateful later.

Much of my parents' help was simply part of trying to understand my differences. From the age of four, I had a psychiatrist; from the age of 10 or 11, I went with my parents to meetings of the Tourette's Syndrome Association. My parents have read hundreds of books about my disorders, listened to my remarks about my difficulty fitting in, given me advice on how to deal with frustrating peers, and helped me cultivate friendships with those who seemed to understand me.

My parents learned volumes of information about the conditions I have, but most of all, they learned who I am.

My dad is a hematologist, treating people with blood diseases like leukemia and hemophilia. Besides working directly with patients he is a researcher, medical school lecturer, editor of a medical journal, and head of a research ethics committee.

My mom is a doctor of occupational medicine, working with people who make work-injury claims, charting their cases and making decisions about workers' compensation, drugs, and vacation time. As physicians, my parents know perfectly well that knowledge of a diagnosis can help in dealing with a patient. But they understand also that each patient is unique, with idiosyncrasies unrelated to the diagnosis. They understand that Erika as a person comes before Erika as a patient.

They understand me.

Mom and Dad have always supported me in my struggle to come to terms with my Asperger's Syndrome and Tourette's Syndrome, and perhaps they sensed that writing and other forms of artwork play a large role in this struggle. I have learned to understand the rest of the world by writing about it, and when I have been unable to understand it, I have taken refuge in other worlds I've created through writing, painting, and drawing. I cannot remember a time when my creative urges went unindulged.

I demanded entire reams of paper for drawing from the age of two. At that time, my pictures were nothing but shapeless scribbles, but I always got as much paper as I wanted. I remember it well: perfectly white paper in packages of three hundred sheets, enfolded in brown wrapping with the name "Quill" and a picture of a feather pen.

Later I started wanting blank books to write in, and my parents bought me those, too. The books were always the kind with a binding like real hardcover books, sometimes with a beautiful pattern on the front and back covers, sometimes with a picture on the front. I liked especially the extra-small ones.

Sometimes I filled the books to the last page with stories from my imagination; sometimes I only got about halfway through the book with writing and filled the rest with drawings. Once I took scissors to a book and painstakingly cut a rectangle out of the center of each page, so that when the book was closed, there was a secret empty space inside it where I could hide small treasures. If my parents saw any of my uses of blank books as wasteful, they kept it to themselves.

When I became a teenager and started hoping to publish a book, my parents didn't let me down. Mom would take me to her office to make half a dozen copies of my manuscripts at once, and let me have all the envelopes and stamps I needed for sending them off.

Of course, now that I look back on those writings, I know that they never could have been published, and that if they had, they would have embarrassed me forever. Mom must have known that, but she let me learn for myself.

Besides indulging my artistic impulses, my parents discovered and accepted my unusual style of learning. Early in my life, they tried punishments to control me: time-outs, spankings, revoking of privileges. Soon, however, they found that I was like a cat rather than a dog. Instead of seeing punishment as an unpleasant consequence to be avoided by changing my behavior, I saw it as a malicious attack, against which I had to retaliate.

No amount of lecturing could change my angry reaction, so my parents learned to live with it. Mom noticed, for example, that as a small child I found it calming to be held tightly. She would soothe my rages in that way, enduring the outrage of onlookers who thought she was rewarding my violence by hugging me.

Mom was especially helpful with school problems, and I certainly needed the help. My teachers in grade school either hated me or loved me. If they couldn't stand anything unexpected, they hated me, and if they couldn't stand being bored, they loved me. Luckily I got quite a few of the latter type, but I still wound up in some classes where I drove the instructors absolutely crazy.

As I said earlier, when I corrected my kindergarten teachers' grammar, the school's response was to send a note to my mother, demanding that she come in for a day and see what an awful kid I was. She came in for a day and saw, in her opinion, what an awful school it was, and soon I moved to a different one.

When I was 18 and Macalester College was reviewing my application, I received a message asking about the fact that I had been a member of no sports teams or school clubs. Instead of scraping up the few things I had done that vaguely suggested a social life and putting an exaggeratedly positive spin on them, my mother and I decided to be honest. We each wrote an essay for the college describing my disorders.

I was an A and B student; my SAT score was 800 on the verbal part and 580 on the math. Macalester turned me down. The official reason: I had once gotten a C in chemistry, in my junior year, as an end-of-the-second-trimester grade, three months before I finished the year with a B in that class.

Mom was outraged. She contacted the authorities at Macalester, argued to have me accepted, complained fiercely when they refused, and finally assured me that I was better off going to Augsburg College.

Life Skills

The girl left Spanish class. On her way out her teacher congratulated her. "Otra calificación perfecta! Another perfect grade, sí? Are you going to be a translator, señorita?"

"Of course I'm going to be a translator. I've always wanted to be a translator."

"Muy bién! Una traductora! Sabes qué es una traductora? Do you know what a traductora is?"

"Sí. Una mujer que traduce." The girl looked at her for another moment, then repeated her answer in English. The teacher did not notice the parody of her own condescending voice. "A woman who translates. I'll be late for my bus, Señora."

"Muy bién. Hasta mañana!"

No one else said anything to the girl as she passed the other students leaving the class and headed for her locker.

An A+ on her test, as usual. She didn't rejoice. She didn't remember ever seeing any grade other than an A+ in that classroom. Certainly none of the other students ever showed her their tests. They never even looked at her, except with open mouths and wary eyes when she was "having a spazz," or with smirking faces when they were playing a joke, telling her Ricky, or Daniel, or whoever, was in love with her and she ought to go kiss him. They looked at the too-small T-shirt that she didn't know she was supposed to put a bra under, and they looked at the big pink sweatpants that she didn't know had never been in style, and they looked at the face that she didn't know was supposed to have makeup on it, and they didn't look *at her*. Or at the A+ on her Spanish test.

Other students didn't notice the A+. They noticed the dancing on the teacher's desk when she'd forgotten her medication, and they noticed the stories passed down since grade school that she used to bite people. Somehow they hadn't figured out, in the three years they'd been writing fake love letters here at Northside Junior High, that she no longer responded to that. They hadn't figured out that she'd spent all of grade school learning that people were insensitive, especially to someone clueless enough to take so long to learn that simple fact about humanity. They hadn't figured out that, even though she still didn't know how to tell a fake love letter from a real one—because she'd never seen a real one—she understood that no love letter anyone wrote to her would ever be real.

She got to her locker. Her locker was right next to the Life Skills Office. Every school has to come up with its own euphemism for Special Ed, she thought, watching Miss Colleen, the social worker, make a note on a whiteboard just inside the Life Skills Office's open door.

Miss Colleen was overweight. The girl had noticed that most Life Skills staff members were female and overweight. Maybe they had been unpopular in their childhood, too. Maybe they wanted to help people who had gone through the same pain they had. It was similar pain, except that Life Skills students usually were *gifted* and Life Skills staff members usually were *stupid*,[2] and didn't know how to help the people they chose to help. They thought that having a mental disability meant having the mind of a three-year-old. The girl had the mind of a 40-year-old, but she was part of Life Skills, so nobody ever noticed.

She turned the dial on her lock. She remembered the combination. She took out her coat and her boots, then shut her locker door and looked up and saw Miss Colleen looking down on her.

"How do we shut our lockers?" Miss Colleen said.

What did she mean? Was she asking the girl a question about lockers? Did she want advice? What was the girl supposed to say?

---

[2] There are some very talented Special Education teachers, but this is how I felt at 14. Painful as it is, it's a valuable perspective!

"How do we shut our lockers?" repeated Miss Colleen, now slightly annoyed.

Then the girl understood what she meant. I must have shut my locker too loudly, she thought in exasperation. Damn it! She wants me to say *quietly.* Or *softly.* The girl's teeth tightened. Miss Colleen, she said silently, do you know that I could say one hundred words by the time I was one year old? Do you know that I could spell better than you when I was five? Do you know that I am fluent in German and Spanish and scored 153 on my IQ test and nevertheless have no friends and have to deal with an average of one fake love letter per month and do not need this right now?

Miss Colleen didn't know. Miss Colleen would never know. She only knew that she'd had to ask the girl twice how she should have shut her locker, and that the girl hadn't answered, and, having the mind of a three-year-old, as she knew all Life Skills children did, probably hadn't understood the question. She repeated it, very slowly, enunciating the words with ultimate clarity, *"How do we shut our lockers?"*

We! How do we shut our lockers! The girl was by now struggling visibly to keep her temper. She'd heard of the royal "we", implying the first person singular; now there must be a Life Skills "we" implying the second person, and she didn't like it. If she just said "quietly," she could put on her coat and her boots and get down to Bus Number 17 exactly on time and be at home doing her Spanish in under 10 minutes. But she couldn't say "quietly" because she felt so degraded that her mouth wouldn't open because her teeth were clenched together so hard, and she wanted to scream! What was Miss Colleen doing now, damn it?

Miss Colleen was leaning over the girl with her lips in a little round O-shape, as if she were about to kiss her, but instead she was making a sound, clearly, distinctly, so as to leave no doubt whatsoever in the little three-year-old's mind as to what she was doing:

"Qu Qu Qu "

Like Aunt Barb. Like Aunt Barb when Cousin Max was 11 months old and she was trying to get him to say "boat." She was prompting her. She was prompting her with the first syllable of "quietly." She honestly thought the girl didn't know what she wanted her to say, and she was prompting her.

The girl's teeth were clamped together so hard she felt that they were going to break. Instead, they opened.

And she bit Miss Colleen.

My Journey

The prefix *auto* means "self," so *autism* is the condition of being by oneself, being alone. The name is so appropriate that two scientists, discovering autism independently and simultaneously in different parts of the world, both named it autism.

Asperger's Syndrome, which I have, often is considered a form of autism. Tourette's Syndrome, which I have also, is characterized by impulse-control problems and by involuntary movements and vocalizations called tics, though mine have calmed with maturity and been controlled with medications.

Associated with my Tourette's Syndrome and Asperger's Syndrome are some other conditions. I have mild obsessive-compulsive disorder (OCD). I have some symptoms similar to those of attention deficit disorder (ADD) and attention deficit hyperactivity disorder (ADHD), although those may just be symptoms of my Asperger's and Tourette's. All of these are things I have had to come to terms with through a struggle lasting many years.

People with Asperger's Syndrome do not fit into the society around them. We do not instinctively pick up clues in body language and voice tone that tell us what people mean. We do not know automatically how to make friends; we have to study at it for years. We are socially inept until we have learned, sometimes over a lifetime, how to function in society.

We seldom have below-average intelligence. I do not want to perpetuate the myth that all autistics can accomplish huge mathematical feats in their heads, but the fact is that many do have some startling talent, as do people with Tourette's.

Yet one is expected to be ashamed of having Tourette's, autism, or any sort of other mental or emotional disability. When I break the rule and discuss my disorders as openly as my race or gender, some people become embarrassed and uncomfortable. Other people admire me, thinking that it must take immense courage to talk about such things. But for me, my mental conditions are not taboo; they are just part of who I am.

Tourette's and Asperger's are more common in men than in women, so as a woman with both, I am a member of an invisible minority. With my disorders piled on top of my gender and my age, I belong to a group so small that few people have reason to think about it.

Many things are easier for me than for those with more severe Tourette's or autism. Sometimes, when pleading their case to the normal people who misunderstand them, I feel as if I am standing up for the rights of a race with whom I share a part of my heritage—a multiracial woman and one with a mild disorder experience a taste of what their more strongly affected sisters do. Knowing the normal world more intimately than many autistics know it, I may even make a good link between the two realities.

Other children feared, mocked, and took advantage of my disabilities throughout grade school. They, and many of my teachers, modeled their opinions of me after some preconceived concept of abnormality. They saw that I was different, heard that I had a mental diagnosis, and looked no further.

In addition, the authorities were always punishing me. This was not for my lack of trying to behave well. To nearly the best of my ability, I did what I was told.

Autistic children usually have no desire to be dishonest, and I wasn't an exception. I avoided skipping class, drawing on the walls, cheating on assignments, and breaking even the minor rules I found stupid, like the no-hats-no-jackets policy, or the rule in high school that underclassmen couldn't go off-campus during school hours. I was unwilling to glance over at a classmate's book to see what page we were on, because we had been told not to look at each other's work.

Ironically, I got suspended more often than most of my peers, because I had no knowledge of social rules and ended up offending and frightening people when trying to get a laugh out of them. I couldn't manage the nuances that made the difference between a joke and a threat or insult.

The main features of my Tourette's syndrome were severe impulsive behavior and a volatile temper. I did things like walking up and kissing classmates on the neck without warning, and I could get into physical fights over an insect's species.

When asked why I'd done something, I could never explain it. It had just happened. Even though I avoided deliberate transgressions that were a part of everyday life for other students, I often broke rules by accident or in the heat of the moment. The principal's office became one of the most familiar places in the school.

I learned to speak, read, and write very early, and have continued to develop those abilities. There were people who admired me for being so successful with words despite my Asperger's and Tourette's. Yet this success was not despite my disorders, but because of them. Some autistic people are mathematical prodigies; I was a linguistic prodigy. Whatever my mental conditions took from me, they gave me facility with words and language.

While the field of language was my strong suit, the field of social interaction was not. I had a few friends, but most of my interpersonal contact involved people trying to get me to do something stupid so they could laugh at me. I usually did it. I craved attention so much that, even when not egged on, I did whatever ridiculous things came into my head, just so people would laugh and remind me that I existed.

My internal life was extremely active. I put on little puppet shows for myself with my hands, pretending they were ducks and swans and dogs and monsters that acted out complicated dramas. I made up stories and told them to myself while wandering around the playground. I learned not to care about the strange looks I got from other kids. During some stages of my childhood, I even took a kind of weird pleasure in being an outcast, able to scare people away just by looking at them.

I knew that human culture places great value on physical appearance. My first mistake was thinking that I could win popularity by beauty alone. My second was expecting that I could manage the complicated codes of what beauty was. I wore tight, low-necked shirts, but didn't know I was supposed to wear anything under them. I wore lots of makeup—too much, and the wrong colors. I had no idea what went with what. And even when I did manage to look beautiful, it didn't make up for being a weirdo. I had the same desire for love and popularity that normal girls had, but it took me a long time to learn to fulfill it.

Throughout my childhood, teens, and young adulthood I struggled to fit in. I asked questions of my parents, teachers, and friends, and told them all the difficulties I had in understanding my classmates. I read books about normal people and books about autistic people. I watched social interaction, trying to figure out how it worked.

Most of all, I wrote. I crystallized my thoughts about the world by keeping a diary. I worked to comprehend humans by exploring and describing them in the written word. I invented and wrote about imaginary cultures to help me understand my own.

And very, very gradually, I *succeeded*.

It has taken me a very long time to learn some of the rules of human interaction, to come to terms with the parts of me that I have not been able to change, and to help other people accept me the way I am. I am not someone who had a disease and cured herself, but someone who was born to think differently. At first I didn't fit into the society of normal humans. Slowly I gained a better understanding of the world and brought the world a better understanding of me.

Crazy

She sat on the hearthstone of the fireplace, in the student lounge. It was only a foot high, but high enough to sit on. It was slightly uncomfortable, but that didn't bother her, not in the mood she was in: happy, full of energy, done with classes for the day, even with homework. And two full hours behind her medication schedule.

"And in biology class, we talked about hormone cycles. Who would've expected that a woman's estrogen cycle goes on a monthly basis and a man's testosterone cycle is daily? Think of it, Kris. We must be the only species where the female has her mating season every 28 days and the male has it every 24 hours! No wonder the genders don't get along!" She burst out laughing, her hand repeatedly pushing her golden-brown hair behind her ear and shoving her wire-rimmed glasses up on the bridge of her nose.

Her voice was strident, drawing the attention of a few other students on a nearby couch, but Kristin, sitting next to her, joined her laughter.

"You're right, it's crazy." Kris stretched her legs out in front of her and crossed them at the ankles, careful of her woven ankle bracelets. "Poor guys. Going into heat every day. No wonder they have nothing but sex on their minds. It certainly makes everything a bit more complicated."

"We should just be like plants," her friend continued. "Instead of all these complicated courtship rituals, just set up our sex organs so they attract bugs, and let the bugs carry our genetic material from one person to the other." She clasped her arms around her own bent knees, interlaced her fingers, and began to rock gently. "But then, some other species might come and cut them off and use them in their courtship. I wonder if that's the reason people give each other flowers to express love—because they're the plants' genitals."

Kris shuddered, playing with her bead necklace. "Scary thought." Her nervously added chuckle multiplied her friend's laughter, and the golden-brown hair tossed back and shook in mirth.

"Pollination! Geez! I shouldn't have started this conversation. Now I don't even feel like going outside. I'm allergic to plant sperm." She slid forward until her backside was almost off the hearthstone, and she tipped her grinning face up at the ceiling. "Plants are such perverts." She fell into a torrent of giggles.

Kristin's eyebrows crawled together in concern, while her eyes darted to the side to judge how much notice other people in the lounge were taking of their discussion. "Have you taken your pills?"

"Of course not." She shook with laughter. "Hey! I had a pepper plant once that I pollinated with a paintbrush so it could grow peppers. What do you think, Kris, if I pollinate my plants with a paintbrush, am I having sex with them?" Her eyes widened, and a fresh scream of laughter burst out. "Can they even consent? Is it rape? I'm a plant rapist!"

"That was too loud. You have to calm down. Please." Kristin put a hand on her arm.

A quicker hand threw it off. "Don't touch me! Unwanted physical contact! Careful, or you'll turn into a rapist too!" A sudden leap and she was standing on the hearthstone, a foot above the floor, waving her arms around. "Grab my arm, will you? Right above the elbow! You know, that part of the human arm shouldn't even exist! It should be illegal! Do you know why?"

The room had become very quiet.

"Please. Calm down. You're making people uncomfortable."

"Because it causes deafness! Everyone who has that part of their arm is at a high risk for hearing loss! You know why? Because if you take your shirt off and go like this—" she raised her upper arm and slapped it against her ear, "—it can damage your eardrum! So there!"

Kristin sighed. "Would you please come down from there, and we'll go someplace else?"

"No! I won't come down!" The raised arm dropped to her side, like her other arm, her elbows and knees bent. "I won't come down. I'm going to jump! Really! I'm going to jump! Don't think I won't do it, because I will!" And then she laughed so hard she almost fell.

"All right. Jump down and come back to your dorm and take your pills." Kristin was openly pleading now, with no idea if it was doing any good.

"Stop talking like that! If you had any idea how much I hate that tone of voice. If you had any idea how many special-ed teachers have talked to me that way, how many idiots think that every kid who's a little weird can't understand anything but *baby talk*." Her face was now swollen with rage, her bent arms tense, her fists clenched to bloodless white. "Go away!"

Then she jumped. Kristin saw her spring like an agile animal, saw her hip, her side, her shoulder hit the floor, and her golden-brown head fall limp.

Two or three people got up and hurried out of the lounge.

Kristin knelt beside her. "Oh no. Oh, damn it, are you really hurt? How the hell did that happen? Please tell me you're okay."

"No, I'm dead as a doornail. Get off me. You're disturbing the peace of my soul." Narrowed eyes, snarling grin; hysterical laughs rang out like coughs. Two hands shot out and grabbed Kristin's collar. "*I'mmm the ghoooost of the stuuuudeeent looouuunge fiiireplaaace.*" Another convulsion of laughter—hands reaching up and catching the blue fabric of Kristin's shirt, twisting and shaking.

Snap!

Silence. They froze, as eyes behind wire-rimmed glasses assessed the damage. Other people tried to look away. Beads bounced with delicate clicks across the floor.

"I broke your necklace."

"It's okay." Forced calmness contended with concern.

"I broke it. I can't believe I did that." She pushed herself to her feet. "I have to get out of here. I'm going crazy." A swift brush of hair out of a panicked face. "I'm so sorry. Damn it." Rushing for the door, face flushed in shame. "I have to go."

"Do you need me to walk back to your dorm with you?"

"No. I'll just go back there, take my pills and go to bed. Damn it! I'm so sorry."

The door to the lounge swished shut and footsteps thumped down the hall until Kristin couldn't hear them anymore. Sighing, she bent down again and began to pick up beads and bits of string. She knew she'd never been in any real danger, and that even the broken necklace was an accident, unplanned even by the insanity. Within a week she knew she'd find a package in her mailbox, and the necklace inside would perhaps be longer, perhaps have brighter beads than the one that had broken.

Would that bring peace of mind? Would there still be moments, years from now, when her friend's head would lean forward into hands that clenched in the golden-brown hair, longing to erase the memory? Did each of the hundreds of similar memories build up like an unsteady wall of shame that leaned against the conscience?

Kristin would never know. No matter how much she cared for them, there were some people she had given up trying to understand.

Unmedicated

I take three pills in the morning and two in the evening. Of the morning pills, one is to keep me awake and help me pay attention. One is to stop panic attacks, one is to keep me from being hyperactive and impulsive, and twitching and fidgeting with Tourette's tics.

One of the evening pills is a second dose of the pill for tics and impulses, the other is to help me sleep. Without the sleeping pill I stay awake until noon the next day. I've never learned to put myself to sleep by imagining dull, repetitive things like sheep jumping over a fence, because for me they aren't dull and repetitive. When I picture something happening in my head, it happens strangely, especially when I'm tired. The sheep are all different colors, or they wear swimsuits and sunglasses. They don't clear the fence; they hit their heads on it, or scrape their bellies and bleed.

If my friends and family were asked what my medicines were for, they would probably think first of my attacks of impulsive behavior. That's the first thing that starts to show when I am late to medicate myself. When I start giggling crazily and saying irrelevant, ludicrous things, my loved ones turn to me and say, "Erika, have you had your meds?"

Not long ago at a family gathering, I waited a few hours to take my pills, afraid that if I took them at the usual time I would fall asleep before it was time to go home. The result was insanity.

I became not just silly, but crude. I pinched people on the behinds. I made loud speculations about the sex lives of Star Trek characters.

"On my next trip," I shouted, "I want to go to Saginaw Bay! Because if the Great Lakes are a picture of a wolf, and Lake Superior is his head, and Lake Michigan is his paw, and Lake Huron is his body, do you know what part of him Saginaw Bay is?"

My family, accustomed to such things, ignored me until I tired myself out, went into a corner by myself, read a book, and calmed down.

That's a fairly typical episode, although they are not always in such bad taste. Sometimes I just get mildly silly, within the range that friends can laugh at pleasantly.

There have also been worse episodes. One semester I took an apple from a student and threw it at the wall; picked up a chair and threatened another student with it; wrapped myself around a third student and started mauling his neck in front of the entire class and the professor; and barricaded myself in the computer room, shouting to people who asked if I needed anything, "Send Kevin in here with a leather bodice and a whip! I require it to survive!"

Finally the madness built so high it broke over the rocks of my own shock and outrage, and I ran home before I could do anything more. In the days afterwards, I was miserably ashamed and depressed, and completely avoided contact with other people.

Such severe outbursts happen less often now than they used to. Of my memories of grade school, over half are memories of being punished for going crazy. Back then I made fewer obscene comments, but I chased and kissed other children all the time, not caring what gender they were or if I even liked them. I mooned people. Once I went through the hallways seizing male students by the arm at random and saying, "Darling, where shall we go on our honeymoon?" The most common answer was "What the f-k?" I wrote their responses in a notebook, and told people I was doing a scientific study.

People are more understanding now than they were when I was a kid. Teachers ask me what the problem is and how they can help, rather than punishing me. Friends are uncomfortable during my insanity, but later when I say I'm sorry, they accept my apology and seem more concerned than offended. Apparently adults can get away with more than children can.

During the attacks of hyperactivity, I crave attention and laughter from other people, but if they do laugh, I get more hyperactive. My closest friends know that I calm down faster if I'm ignored. It also helps to go somewhere alone for a while and do something solitary like reading. Of course, the first thing to do is to take my pills.

Panic attacks usually start with a legitimate inconvenience. For example, something goes wrong with my computer, or the school bureaucracy is uncooperative with my attempts to pay tuition bills or sign up for a dorm.

However, it's not always something that would get me truly upset at a good time. Once I had a panic attack when I couldn't get a menu on my computer to be in the part of the screen where I wanted it. Sometimes small things trigger panic attacks, and sometimes they don't. I don't know what makes the difference, but pills have a big part in it.

When a panic attack starts my muscles tense up and my breathing becomes fast and tight. Those are typical symptoms of anxiety, but for me, they are a warning sign; I know that soon things will get worse. My breathing rate becomes faster, and it can accelerate so much that it's hard to stop. I start to feel a tingling around the corners of my face, and people tell me that I'll faint if I don't calm down. But if I try to breathe more slowly, I feel that I'm not getting enough air and the panic builds higher.

I start crying uncontrollably. Despair sets in. I feel that everything's going wrong, that nothing will ever work out, that the worst-case scenario will undoubtedly come to pass. Every time someone expresses a hope that something good may happen, or suggests how things might be made better, I come up with some reason why that couldn't possibly work.

I become unreasonably angry, snapping at people who offer help. Then I swing abruptly into remorse, apologize, curse myself, and minutes later begin snapping again.

Even though I know that my panic is hurtful to others, I crave company, becoming still more depressed when people leave me. Then, once alone, silently I curse those people for not caring about me, not wanting to be with me.

I become sensory-defensive. Loud noises, bright lights, and strong smells raise my panic to unbearable levels. Although I don't want to be alone, I can't stand being touched, or even having other people too close to me. It feels like an invasion, like an attack. Sometimes my skin becomes so sensitive that physical contact is actually painful.

The feeling isn't confined to people. There are times when I am so sensitive that even wearing clothing hurts, and there are times when I need my personal space so much that I can't endure being in a small or cluttered room.

There's no clear pattern to what will stop a panic attack. Sometimes, when the initial problem is resolved, the panic begins to wind down slowly. Sometimes it disappears unexpectedly, for no apparent reason. Sometimes I cry myself to sleep and wake up calmer.

As with the impulsive outbursts, though, there's less chance of a panic attack beginning in the first place if I have taken my pills on time. If I haven't, and one does start, the first remedy is to take them as soon as possible.

The tics involved with Tourette's Syndrome are different for each person who has it. Some hit or throw things uncontrollably; some spit or grind their teeth or lick their lips; some yell out words, or repeat what they or other people have said.

I've had several different tics, usually not severe ones but enough to make life difficult. As a young child, I had one noticeable vocal tic. It was *palilalia*: repeating the beginnings of words and sentences several times before finishing them.

My motor tics were many and varied. I shifted my feet back and forth, over and over again, in a repeated pattern; I rubbed my hand briefly and repetitively at my head or my face or my arm; I sucked my thumb much longer than most children.

Now, as a young adult, I have milder tics. There is a distinctly "Touretty" pattern to the way I adjust my glasses and my hair. Sometimes I put the side of my finger to my nostrils and exhale sharply, or raise my upper lip until it rests almost against my nose and breathe on it.

Right now, lying on my stomach on my bed as I write, I am pushing my foot against the top of the footboard in such a way as to force it in between my toes. I have been doing this over and over again without thinking. As with any tic, I could control it for a while if I tried, but as soon as I stopped consciously thinking about controlling it, it would begin again.

A problematic urge is my habit of picking at my skin. I'm not sure if it's a tic or part of my obsessive-compulsive disorder. It started with my discovery of pimples in adolescence. I have never been able to leave them alone, and now I don't even wait for them to become visible. I go over my skin for a quarter-hour or more, usually the skin of my face or chest, squeezing at every tiny irregularity in case there might be a bit of pus or oil in it.

I pick those spots until they become scabs, I pick the scabs until they become scars, and then I open up the scars and start over again. I go through phases: sometimes my chest and my face get a chance to heal, sometimes I spend weeks looking as if I had chicken pox.

The tic that causes me the most problems lately is holding my breath. The urge is similar to the urge to yawn, and indeed the action is very much like a yawn: I lean back, stretch, and take a fast, deep breath. But I hold that breath much longer than the one taken in a regular yawn. So long, in fact, that I begin to lose consciousness.

It seldom gets to the point that I fall down. Usually I just become less aware of my surroundings until I have been breathing again for a while. People watching me usually don't notice anything. Either I go very still, or start shifting slightly as though uncomfortable. My other tics become more severe during these fainting spells, and I may push at my glasses or my hair, or fidget with my feet more rapidly and energetically than usual.

The only thing sure to catch observers' attention is the short, hard exhalation when I let out the breath. However, if people happen to ask me something before I fully come back to consciousness, they will certainly notice that I don't reply, or I'll murmur incoherently or answer inappropriately.

At a party, I was talking with my young cousins, and my cousin Peter said, "The best way to do a maze is to start at the end."

For most mazes, this is true. I have done them that way many times, and I've occasionally tried the challenge of designing a maze that was as hard to go through backwards as forwards.

However, when I heard Peter's comment, I was just coming out of a fainting spell, and somehow the phrase "start at the end" sounded like complete nonsense to me. I burst out laughing, thinking that he had said something ridiculous.

Another time, while having a fainting spell in biology class, I heard the professor end a sentence: "... it's a useful ability for a mammal to have."

I blurted out, "Why? Does it help make milk or something?"

The rest of the class laughed, and it wasn't until I heard more of the discussion that I realized he had been talking about the ability to control bowel movements.

During these attacks, I can have any number of interesting sensations. My skin tingles and my vision is affected. Sometimes it just gets cloudy, and sometimes it goes black entirely. Sometimes my vision remains but I lose the ability to attach meaning to what I see, perceiving only colors and shapes.

Occasionally I have distinct hallucinations. Sometimes they are of things I have seen or thought about recently, like beads when I have been making bead jewelry, or flowers when I have been gardening. Sometimes they're completely unexpected things, like a neon-colored, fuzzy cartoon bird, or a gray-green face covered with tentacles. Sometimes they're just geometric patterns, complicated and multicolored.

One or more of my senses—hearing or smell, for example—may become less sensitive, or disappear for the interim. Or one or another of my senses might become more sensitive, so that I notice the rushing of water in a pipe in the wall, or the quiet ticking of a clock across the room, or the smell of my own sweat, none of which I would notice in full consciousness.

A limb might go limp and heavy for awhile. Sometimes one entire side of my body is affected, and I know for a moment what it might be like to be paralyzed on the right or the left. I might get an erroneous idea of what position my body is in; I may think that I'm sitting when I'm lying down, or that my hand is in my lap when it's on my desk. Sometimes these thoughts even apply to my clothes. I believe for a moment that I'm wearing socks when I'm not, or that my shirt is on backwards when it's on forwards.

All sorts of strange thoughts might come to me, not always related to my body. Sometimes I have *déja vu*. Sometimes I make a strange connection between an aspect of my fainting spell and a topic that has been on my mind. For example, I notice that I am breathing in a pattern of three short breaths at a time, and connect that to the fact that I am taking three classes each day that semester.

Often a nonspecific scenario comes into my head that has no connection to my own life. *Someone wants something and cannot get it.* Or, *There are two ways to do something, and one of them is better than the other.*

Sometimes, when I am having a panic attack, it ends during a fainting spell, or one that has ended begins again. Sometimes, I have inspirations.

Obviously, with so much going on in my mind, my fainting spells distract me from things that need my attention. They are most common when I am sitting still and not physically participating in anything, and so they frequently interrupt when I try to listen in class. On a bad day I miss 30 seconds of the lecture every two or three minutes. I don't know how I continue to get good grades.

There was a phase some years ago when the spells frequently involved convulsions and loss of balance. My body would start jerking uncontrollably and I'd fall to the floor or ground. Sometimes I'd hit myself on things, getting painful bruises. Neurologists and cardiologists studied those fainting spells and found no explanation or treatment. Luckily, the phase ended by itself.

At the moment, the most troublesome part of fainting spells is the increased tic activity during them. Not only do I touch my hair and twitch my feet, I move air around in my mouth and respiratory passages in such a way that it goes up my salivary ducts and sinuses, causing sore cheeks and headaches.

Worst of all, I grind my teeth. Seeing how quickly I have worn through my first few protective retainers, I wonder how I am going to afford dentist bills if this goes on for the rest of my life.

I don't know exactly how well the pills repress the breath-holding tic, but I am fairly sure it happens more when I take the pills late. I will continue trying to find a tic medication that controls the tics better.

At different times in my life I've taken different pills. At first it was only one kind; at other times it has been as many as seven or eight. My psychiatrist and parents have always come up with the ideas for what I will take, based on conversations with me and with each other.

I have no idea how any of the pills work. I'm the poet in my family, the dreamer, the artist, what my brother calls a "literature bum." He is the math and science expert. The concepts of chemistry fascinate me, but whenever I've tried to study the details, I've gotten hopelessly confused.

Certainly, I have no understanding of how the chemicals in those particular medications affect the biology of my brain. I know myself as a person, not as a diagnosis. I don't claim to comprehend the inner biological workings of my disabilities, only the effects they have on my life. I know that when I miss one of the pills, I can't sleep at night; when I miss another, I get drowsy in the day and can't pay attention; when I miss a different one, I have more panic attacks, and so on.

Sometimes I think that maybe I've gotten too used to taking the pills, too dependent on them. If I go two days without them, I have panic attacks in which I become so shaky that it's like having convulsions. That never happened before I took the pills. But I was a small child when I started. My brain and my body have changed since then.

Of course I'd like to be able to live a happy life without medications. I will have to find a time when I have the freedom to risk inconvenient behavior changes, and the courage to risk the emotional trauma that would go with those changes. I would have to cut down slowly, over a long time, and be willing to stop cutting down if it didn't work. I might do it, someday, but for now my pills are too helpful to give up.

Butterfly

Day camp. The unbounded energy of being seven years old. The ability to rise to heights of excitement from finding a frog, riding a horse, making a lanyard bracelet.

And of course, the torment of hearing great quantities of nonsense, both from counselors and from other campers. "Those fish in the lake, they're bullheads. If one of them bites you, you'll die within a day. There's no cure." Or, "We put a special chemical in the swimming pool. If you pee in there, a big red circle will form around you. If you don't believe me, just try it."

Nature hour. Sitting in a circle on the floor of a garage-shaped building in a field, with a curly-haired lady talking to us. "One of the kinds of insects you'll find here at camp is spiders," she lilts, with the air of someone imparting great knowledge to the next generation.

Inevitably, my voice: "Spiders aren't insects. They're arachnids."

"Erika, we don't interrupt. Wait your turn to talk."

"Spiders have eight legs! Insects have six!"

"They are a kind of insect."

My mouth contorts, blood pounds in my brain, the familiar itching begins in my limbs and face that means they are crying out to crush something, hit someone, bite someone. I throw my head back in despair and clench my hands in a futile attempt to ease the ache of staying still, of not climbing over the other campers to attack the nature teacher.

Another day: learning about young animals. "And what do we call a baby rabbit?"

I know the answer. I've read it. The word rabbit breeders use: kitten, the same as the word for a baby cat.

"Nope, that's wrong, Erika. Someone else?"

Rage, like panic, sudden and unbearable. I was right, and she brushed me off as if I had said something pointless. I feel the grimace crawl across my face, looking like crying, tensing my muscles. Through the roar in my head, I hear another child give the answer she wanted: bunny.

Twisting my body from side to side, shifting from one sitting position to another, as if I could find an arrangement of my arms and legs that would stretch the violent urge out of them, even for a moment.

"Sit still, Erika," I hear.

In the field by the forest, a group of us building a campfire. A butterfly sails by, lands, takes off again, flies around us. A butterfly about the size of the circle I can make with my thumb and index finger. Dull brown and gray, but intricately patterned, to camouflage well on a piece of tree bark. It is moving so slowly and so close to us that I have even seen its antennae.

"Look, a butterfly!" I announce.

"It's a moth," says another girl. She is prettily dressed and has well-combed, shoulder-length blond hair.

"No, it's a butterfly," I insist. My voice already has a quality of urgency to it. I am not thinking of the rage that will be on me in a few seconds, but soon I will be able to think of nothing else.

"Butterflies have colors. Moths are really dull brown, like that one."

"Moths have antennae like feathers! That's a butterfly; it has knobs on the ends of its antennae!"

"No, it's a moth."

I call to the counselor in desperation, the anger already starting to take me over. He is so much older than I am; he must know that butterflies have knobs on their antennae. "Look, is that a moth or a butterfly?"

My idea of what adults know is an overestimation. "I have no idea," he calls back. "I guess it's probably a moth."

"See, I was right," says the girl.

My fist crashes violently against her shoulder. The relief of feeling the collision is incredible, a primal pleasure, pure physics. Energy, built up to breaking point, finally directed and released, reverberating through her body and out into the universe. I stagger back from her, already relaxing, but recognizing the beginning of a different kind of anxiety. The counselor is coming over to see what's going on.

Later, sitting in the counselors' office, I watch a different member of the staff prepare a note to my parents. She has written my name "Erica."

"It's spelled with a K," I say.

"Huh." She scrutinizes the paper. "Well, I sure thought it was an E."

She goes into the next room. I puzzle over her words. What did she mean, an E?

I find out soon. She returns with the note. My name reads "Krica."

Anger surges up, memory fades out. Years later I will not recall whether I managed to control myself this time.

With all the teasing I got from peers, all the commands I had to follow from teachers and parents, untruth was the only thing that could bring my seven-year-old mind to that level of fury. I couldn't stand to see reality misrepresented through dishonesty or stupidity, especially by people in positions of power, the people I expected to be honest and intelligent.

When I was punished for doing something I knew was unacceptable I might be defiant, but I knew I was wrong. I reached the boiling-over state, in which the need to hurt someone was a physical pain in itself, only when something untrue was accepted as true. It didn't matter if it were an accusation of something I didn't do, a mis-classification of an animal, or merely an incorrect spelling of my name.

Prodigy

My parents can't remember the first word I ever said. They just have a bunch of pages of words I said in my first year of life. There are over a hundred words in the list; half of them are in German.

Relatives tell me stories of things I said as a baby. Riding a cable car at the state fair, I looked out the window and commented, "People walking way down there." Playing with ribbons, I made up a rhyme: "Ribbons, ribbons, like a bow; we can put them together, oh!"

Early on, pronouns confused me; I called myself "you" because that was what everyone else called me. The grammatical error contrasted strangely with my eloquence. Complaining about being unable to reach the closet doorknob, I said, "You so small, cannot open the door, go in the closet, see all the hangers overhead."

Mom and Dad found that I could memorize sentences quickly and flawlessly, even as a two-year-old. Being fun-loving eccentrics, they taught me to recite how exhaust goes through the innards of a car. When they brought me along to the garage to get their own vehicles repaired, I could perform for the mechanics: "And then it goes into the exhaust manifold, and then it goes into the catalytic converter ... "

I couldn't recite the whole monologue from memory now, but when I could I must have seemed as astonishing as people who can calculate square roots of ten-digit numbers in their heads. I was a psychological curiosity, a verbal savant, but also, to my parents, a lovable child and a great source of fun.

I was just as talkative in my second language. On one of our many trips to Europe, the year I was four we spent a long time waiting for a plane. Finally a stewardess announced in German that those with small children could begin boarding. As my parents started to get up I cried out in protest: "Ich bin nicht *klein*! Ich bin gross und vier!"

The other waiting travelers had heard me talking to my parents in English a few minutes before. They knew I was American, and hadn't expected that an American child would be able to say so fluently in German, "I am not *small*! I am big and four!" Everyone laughed in surprise, and to appease me, my parents waited and boarded with the passengers who had no small children.

On the airplane, I wrote and illustrated a story about a cat eating rats. "Rats! Rats! All to eat!" rejoiced the cat in my English version, and then, when I translated it into German, "Ratten! Ratten! Alle zum Fressen!"

The same year, I was given my first IQ test, and scored in the 150s. One would have expected that I would do well in school, but I had a very short attention span. When I wasn't interested in what was going on, I would often just read a book, or draw or write on a notepad. I didn't grasp the importance of doing schoolwork. I had observed the behavior of my peers and concluded that getting bad grades was not a serious problem, but perhaps was even something of which to be proud.

I had trouble organizing, too. It wasn't easy for me to keep track of what assignments were due when. I always had some project of my own—a story or poem I was writing, or a picture I was drawing—that I didn't want to put down in favor of something like schoolwork.

The only subjects I did well in were the ones I liked: writing and art. When the work was pretty close to what I did in my free time I usually had no trouble getting it done. Sometimes I was unenthusiastic about art or writing classes when I was deeply involved in some poem, story, or drawing of my own, but most of the time those classes interested me enough that I'd set aside my personal projects for them.

Once the teacher took each of us aside at the end of the school year and told us how we had done. I was told that I had come close to failing. I can't remember exactly what she said had prevented that, but I have the impression it was my exceptional work in the artistic and linguistic fields.

As well as being the class weirdo and class clown, I had something of a reputation as the class artist. When my fourth grade acted out *Romeo and Juliet*, a fact briefly mentioned in the 6 PM news, I was widely acclaimed as the best in the play. The few clips of it that were featured on TV included one of my big scenes. In fifth grade, when I was in a school that went up to eighth grade, I won the schoolwide spelling bee, and placed high enough in the district-wide level that I went on to the citywide one.

By junior high I had gained actual interest in how I did in my classes. By the middle of high school I frequently did my homework without parental encouragement and paid at least polite attention in all my classes.

Now that I'm in college, I am conscientious about schoolwork. I might procrastinate sometimes, and ignore or lightly scan reading assignments that don't seem vital to my grade, but I do all the necessary work, almost always on time.

I have gotten only one grade lower than a 3.5 in the 34 classes I've taken so far. My concern for my grades has become strong enough to overcome difficulties I've had with paying attention, keeping organized, and restricting my projects to leisure time.

Language comes to me easily, and so does the process of forming it into arguments. As a young teenager I could take up the most ridiculous opinions and argue for them so logically that no one could find a defense against me, even though they knew the opinions were ridiculous.

I lived with my aunt for a while, and she was always very good to me, but we argued about every little insignificant thing. We had a bitter feud over how unhealthy MSG is. I considered it fairly harmless, but she considered it so bad that, for a while, she would not buy any food that contained it.

I came to my aunt triumphantly one day, saying that I had done some research that supported my opinion.

She was suspicious. "What kind of research?"

"I asked my parents."

My aunt knew that I had the same opinion as my parents on this subject. "That's a rather biased source."

"Well, where can I find a source that isn't biased?" I replied.

She could find no argument against that.

We were riding in the car another day, listening to the song "Imagine" by John Lennon. I commented that it was an antireligious song. She disagreed. A fierce argument followed, and I stuck stubbornly to my interpretation, refusing to concede even the slightest possibility that another one might be valid.

After several minutes she cried exasperatedly, "You always think your opinions are right!"

Laughing as if she had said something ludicrous, which I seriously believed she had, I retorted, "Well, if I didn't think they were right, they wouldn't be my opinions, would they?"

For which there was also no answer.

I argued vehemently against the curfew law. The idea that people under a certain age could not even legally be outside after a certain hour was outrageous to me.

"Why?" I asked. "It can't be to protect children from criminals who might be out at night, because we don't restrict other vulnerable people, like the elderly and the handicapped. A lot of 12-year-olds can defend themselves better than a lot of 80-year-olds. But it would be completely unacceptable to make 80-year-olds stay inside at night, so why do we do it to kids?"

Nobody could think of a defense against that, but nobody agreed with me, either.

"Or is it because young people commit more crimes at night than adults do? That can't be the reason either, because we don't put a curfew on other groups that have higher crime rates. Men, for example! Men commit a whole lot more violent crimes than women or children. Why do we allow them out at night?"

My girlfriends laughed and said I was right, though I could tell they didn't mean it seriously.

"And if there are ethnic groups that have high crime records, it's because they're forced into social conditions that encourage crime, and they get convicted even when they're not guilty because the courts are prejudiced. That's true, but the same could be said of teenagers, couldn't it? Like some racial minorities, we don't have much money of our own, and we have less freedom than other people, and we're stereotyped as being delinquent. So why can't we go out, too?"

The comical part was that I spent my evenings writing and drawing in my room. I didn't even want to go out at night. I just wanted to argue.

I always knew I was gifted in the use of words, and I liked other people to know it. That's one of the ways I antagonized people in my childhood and early teens: they were left with the impression that I cared more about displaying my skills than being modest or staying out of conflicts.

They were quite right, of course. It wasn't until later that I learned the value of the latter two concepts. I was a child who made no excuses for herself, proud and annoying.

In a Future Life

She died,
Struck down by a toxin accidentally poured
In fortune cookie mix,
And lay there
At a cheap funeral
In a small chapel
A nineteen-year-old corpse
Buried in a green satin gown
With a single geranium blossom at her throat
And a bouquet of marigolds between her and the altar
While college girls in black
Spaghetti strapped
Gap dresses
Smeared tears
On bare arms quivering with sobs.

... "So the annotation on it is on Friday? You'll have to get working on it then. Late papers ruin your grade right before finals. You said it was about rhyme? And alliteration? That you have to write, I mean? I don't see any rhymes in the poem."

"I wonder," said Desiree, "if Madame Christina Gray, B.A., Ph.D., became one of the most prominent poets of the 21st century for the purpose of having high school students and their mothers fret about when annotations on her work are due, which of her brilliant techniques they're assigned to stare at under a microscope, and whether her poems rhyme." Desiree pushed her backpack and folder across the counter, making more room to lean on her elbows and look down at the poem in her hands.

"That really doesn't matter during finals week," said her mother, smiling sweetly. "Now, you'll have to move your stuff upstairs, honey. But I want to see that annotation written before supper, okay? You're an ace at writing, but don't think you can fall behind in your work and still keep getting all As. C'mon, honey, chop-chop! Get your things upstairs and let me set the table."

Desiree sighed. "It's not a table. It's a counter." She stood up painfully and stared for a moment at the poem standing out darkly in black print against the bright ugly pink of the paper. "I simply have to prepare my faculties for the moral catastrophe of dissecting and analyzing this poor, defenseless little masterpiece so that one teacher's bloated ego can be fed enough that it feels like giving me a good grade."

"Dear me, that's harsh," said her mother, gathering spoons from a drawer.

"Thank you."

Desiree's mother looked up suddenly from her work. "There's something about that poem that really gets to you, isn't there?" she asked, giving her daughter an intrigued look.

"If you mean me, yes. If you intend the word 'you' in its generic sense, meaning any person, including the speaker, then no. Because I can see you don't appreciate it in the least." The forcefully delivered sentence left the room full of a palpable need for a change of subject.

"Oh, I was going to ask you one more thing. Did you find a group of girls to go to the prom with?"

"No. I found a boy! Tall, dark, handsome, intelligent, desperately and passionately in love with me…."

"Oh, really?" Her mother's face lit up.

"Of course not. I can't believe you thought I meant that." Desiree began, slowly, to lift the strap of her backpack up over her shoulder, still poring over the lines of verse in the other hand. "I didn't find any girls either. One group said they'd 'think' about it." The quotation marks were audible in her pronunciation of "think."

"Well, that's good. I'm sure you'll find someone to take you, honey. You're a very pretty girl, you know."

Desiree paused halfway to the stairs, the poem on top of the folder in her left hand, the backpack slung over her right shoulder. "It occurred to me once," she said softly, a strange light in her eyes, "that maybe that was all that mattered. It occurred to me that it was all looks and brains. More looks, less brain, and snap, you're popular! Maybe being popular is all superficial silliness, and maybe people who hang out with popular people are all insufferable, and maybe if I were popular, I would rather die than stay that way. Do you think that's how it is, Mom?"

A long glance at Desiree revealed, to her mother's surprise, that she was serious.

"Of course not, Des," said her mother, forcing a laugh. "And stop making that spooky face, you're giving me the heebie-jeebies."

"I went to a psychiatrist on Thursday," said Tiffany proudly.

"About time," joked Melanie, leaning way over to reach for the egg rolls, and being punished by Providence for this impoliteness by getting soy sauce from her mock duck all over the left breast of her T-shirt. This was not even noticed in the frenzy of the others finding out why Tiffany had gone to a psychiatrist.

"It was one of those ones who hypnotize you," said Tiffany, who had, as usual, finished her meal before anyone else did and was delicately arranging her utensils for easier removal by the waiter. "To find out who you were in another life. I always wanted to be hypnotized. It was a birthday present from Mom and Dad. And I found out I used to be Isaac Asimov."

This was taken with less than wild astonishment and admiration, as no one at the table knew who Isaac Asimov was.

"He was a guy who wrote books," said Tiffany. "More books than anyone. Over 400."

"Science fiction?"

"Yes, I think the doctor said that."

"The Martian Chronicles?"

"I believe he mentioned those."

"Then I know who you're talking about. And you got cheated. Unless you're a lot younger than you look. He died eight years ago, and *Martian Chronicles* was written by Ray Bradbury!" Melanie swallowed the mouthful of rice through which she had just informed her friend of her hypnotist's deceit, and sucked noisily on her root beer for a while. Sophie made a face as though someone were about to kill her, and Melanie very deliberately flicked a drop of root beer off the end of the straw at Sophie's pink-and-white sweatshirt with the 18 teddy bears in the little red shirts with letters on them that spelled out Have a Beary Happy Day.

Sophie squealed, but contented herself with a petulant glare at Melanie and a change of subject. "Do any of you want to know who I was in my last life?"

"No," said Melanie.

"Why not?"

"Because I already know. You were Theodore Roosevelt." Sophie had a crush on Theodore Roosevelt because teddy bears were named after him.

"Nope. Eleanor." Sophie smiled proudly.

"That's interesting. She was married to Franklin Roosevelt."

"Oh." Sophie pouted. "Then never mind."

"I think I was H. W. Fowler," said Lena smugly. "Fowler, the guy the English professor talked about yesterday. Because I always use grammar so good."

Everyone nodded in solemn admiration. Except Melanie, who smirked.

"This is your big day, hon," said Desiree's mother, looking up proudly at the red-gowned girl standing on the garden path. "Dear me, you look terrific in that dress. A regular prom queen. I have to get some pictures before you go."

"Mom?" Desiree looked down at her mother, on all fours in the flowerbed with a handful of weeds, the other hand grasping a trowel.

"Yes, honey?"

"What are those ones?"

"Those what?"

"Flowers. The ones that look like daisies, with the dark brown centers and the orange petals."

"Those are gaillardia. Cheerful-looking things, aren't they? Haven't you seen them before?"

"I've looked at them lots of times, but I guess I'd just never bothered to ask you what they were called."

"Well, they're called gaillardia. Which reminds me, how about your corsage? That dress would look stunning with a rosebud pinned on it, and I just happen to have one on this very bush. Just right, not all open, but beginning to. Shall I cut it for you?"

"No, thank you," said Desiree. "I'd like some of … those other flowers instead."

"Gaillardia? On that dress? It wouldn't match, dear. They're the wrong color, the wrong shape. How about lilies of the valley?"

"Gaillardia," said Desiree, very distinctly. "Orange is my favorite color and I want gaillardia on my dress."

"Well, all right." Looking at her daughter out of the corner of her eye, her mother snipped a small bloom from the patch of sun-color that stood out brightly from the other flowers.

"Are you okay today, hon? You don't seem yourself."

"I am fine," said Desiree. "You know I like orange flowers. I've always liked orange flowers."

"But you don't sound quite like you're happy."

"I had a dream last night," she answered sharply, sliding the stem in through one buttonhole and out another.

"Of course you did, honey," laughed her mother, uprooting a long string of creeping Charlie. "So did I."

"And what was yours? That dreamers often lie?"

"Eh?" Her mother looked up at her curiously. "What do you mean?"

"Nothing."

"Oh, well. What was your dream about, dear? You know I like hearing your dreams. They're always so interesting."

"I think it was a good dream," murmured Desiree, toying with the flower on her chest. "Though I don't remember it too well. I was the most popular person in the school."

"Oh, how charming! What was it like?"

"I don't know," said Desiree thoughtfully. "It's strange, but I can't really remember much about what it was like. You know how dreams are? I can't even remember the fun parts, and that's all that makes a dream worthwhile, anyway. I just recall vaguely that I had a lot of friends, and three really good ones in particular. If I didn't know that I must've had fun, I'd wonder whether I did."

"Oh, well." Her mother went back to weeding. "I'm sure you had a grand time. Maybe it was a prediction for the future. You know how those things sometimes are. Reincarnation and all that. Why, I had a dream once, that it was raining, and then I woke up and what do you know—"

A screeching set of brakes and a chatter of young feminine voices from the open window of a van cut into their conversation.

"Oh, look, honey, there's your ride. Remember to keep an eye on your purse. I'm sure you have enough money in there for dinner; Chinese food never costs too much. Just don't lose any of it. The money, I mean, not the Chinese food! But most of all, have a good time!" She waved enthusiastically as Desiree closed the gate behind her and began to cross the street toward the waiting vehicle.

As she climbed into the back seat, she opened her purse just slightly, not so much to make sure the money was still there as to glance once more at a folded sheet of pink paper that she carried with her.

"You've been laughing at everyone," Tiffany accused, "why don't you tell us who you were?"

"You really want to know?" said Melanie.

"Sure."

"Nobody."

"What? You had to be somebody." Tiffany's eyes narrowed.

"If I was, I don't know it."

"Think about it. All you have to do is find something about you that matches something about someone dead. What's strange about you? What makes you different?"

"I'm a nasty, sloppy pig."

"Oh, no you're not, Melanie honey." Tiffany reached to hug her.

"Yes I am," said Melanie, "and I don't think I ever was anyone but me." She pulled away. "I think this is my first life. But I'm going to be someone."

"Going to? How can you tell that?"

"I don't know. I just know I'm going to have other lives. I mean, what's the point, if my soul's never been used before, why just throw it away? If God's in the habit of recycling, I don't see why I should be his only disposable."

"Oh, Melanie, that was so cute!" giggled Sophie.

"And besides," said Melanie, with the look coming into her eyes that Sophie always called her weird-alien look, "I premember it."

"How can you remember something that hasn't happened yet?" said Lena.

"Not remember. Premember. That's what I call it anyway. I premember all sorts of things that are going to happen to me in a future life."

"I never heard of that before," said Tiffany. "Knowing who you're going to be?"

"Who are you going to be?" said Sophie.

"She's going to be a famous writer, because she's so smart," suggested Lena. Everyone was feeling sorry for Melanie because she'd said she was a nasty pig.

"She's going to be a movie star."

"She's going to be Miss America."

"She's going to be the President."

"I am not," said Melanie indignantly.

"Then who are you going to be?" countered Tiffany.

Melanie finished her last bite of mock duck, probed her teeth with her tongue and found a grain of rice stuck there. She took a gulp of root beer and propelled a tiny stream through the space between two teeth, dislodging the particle. "I am going," she said with dignity, "to be a very ordinary girl, in a high school with about 400 other kids, and they are all going to hate me. They'll tease me about everything they can think of, and finally, when I learn to ignore them, they will start ignoring me and I will be nobody. I seriously doubt that I will even be voted Most Something-or-other at the end of high school, let alone be Miss America."

"That's so sad," said Sophie. There was actually a tear in her right eye.

"You're crazy," said Tiffany. "In other lives you're supposed to be someone famous. Like Isaac Asimov, or Roosevelt, or..."

"Fowler," prompted Lena.

"Yeah. Fowler. You can't be an ordinary kid."

"Who says?"

"Who says?! Did you ever hear about anyone being someone ordinary in another life? Or read about it?"

"Once."

"Where?"

"Shouts and Murmurs."

"What's that?"

"The last page of the *New Yorker*."

"That's the comedy page," said Lena. "The things there are parodies. That means they're not true. We learned in English class last week what a parody is."

"Well, I'm going to be an ordinary kid," said Melanie obstinately, "and nobody is going to like me." She cracked open the fortune cookie in her hand.

"What's your fortune?" said Sophie.

Melanie grinned and crumpled the plastic wrapper, then broke the cookie into smaller pieces for less painful ingestion. "*You will die from eating a poisoned fortune cookie,*" she said. She knew she had the weird-alien look on her and she didn't care.

"No, seriously," said Tiffany. "Seriously, what does it say?"

Melanie rubbed her finger along the broken edge of one of her cookie shards, smoothing it. "'*You will be a 19-year-old corpse in a green satin gown.*'"

"Enough joking," said Tiffany. "What's your fortune?"

"'At a cheap funeral in a small chapel, college girls in black Gap dresses will smear tears across bare arms trembling with sobs.'" Melanie cracked each of her three fortune cookie pieces in two, contemplatively, deliberately, raising the number to six.

"Melanieee," pleaded Sophie. "Stop talking like that. And stop making that face. You look creepy."

Melanie raised her handful of cookie bits a little closer to her mouth. "There'll be a single geranium at my throat," she confided, "and a bouquet of marigolds between the altar and me."

"That's 'between the altar and I,'" corrected Lena inaccurately. "Seriously, what does it say?"

Melanie flinched. "Seriously?" She consulted the slip of paper. "*Your life will be long and prosperous.*" She put all six pieces of cookie in her mouth and crunched happily.

"For a second there you were looking like you hated all of us," said Tiffany wonderingly.

"Hated you?" Melanie smiled. "How could I hate you? You're very normal people. In my future life, I'd do anything to have people like you hang out with me." She sucked the last bits of cookie from between her teeth and grabbed the flower at the center of the table by its head, dragging it out of the vase. "What do you call it when everyone in the United States has a pink car?"

"A pink car nation. Old joke," said Tiffany.

"Besides, that's not a carnation," Sophie added as Melanie slipped the stem into her back pocket, leaving the flower sticking out, a ruffled spot of sunlight on her left buttock. "And it's not pink. It's sort of orangish-reddish."

The waitress came with the check. They split it and walked down the street to the bus stop.

While they were waiting for the bus, Melanie died.

A poet was at her funeral.

Having a Reason

As Polly listened to the assistant principal at Ricki's school, she felt her muscles tense.[1]

"I have no idea what happened, but Ricki kicked another child *again*, and handicap or not, we just can't have that."

Over the years, Polly had spent countless hours smoothing things over after Ricki's violent outbursts, and always, when she thought she had things fixed, smoothed, and assured, Ricki blew up again, shattering people's trust and throwing life into an uproar.

This time, after Ricki had been home for several days, Polly spent a tension-filled hour negotiating desperately with Ricki's teachers and the assistant principal, who was now on the phone, sounding hurt and betrayed.

Ricki had kicked another child, without provocation, after having been back in school for an hour.

Polly led her quiet, sullen daughter out to their old brown station wagon. Both were tense, Ricki looking mostly at the ground. Polly had been crying. What had she done to deserve this? A sigh escaped that was half a sob. Where had she gone wrong? Had she been too angry with Ricki while she'd been home for the last few days? Was this Ricki's revenge?

---

[1] *Author's Note:* My mother contributed to this chapter.

On the other hand, Polly thought, opening the door on her side of the car, maybe she'd been too lax, maybe she'd failed to make Ricki understand how serious things were. When she got mad and talked harshly, Ricki screwed up her face and threw horrible frightening rages.

Polly settled behind the wheel, pulling her seatbelt down and clicking it into the buckle.

Maybe she'd messed up everything from the beginning. She wasn't that strict. Demanding, yes, strict—not with her daughter. Or maybe, because she demanded so much of herself, she'd been too strict with Ricki, demanded too much, and created a sullen, angry girl who saw punishment as the answer to everything. Maybe Ricki felt that now it was her turn to punish the entire world.

Polly put her hands on the wheel. "Why, Ricki?"

She turned the ignition, and nearly started crying again. "Why did you have to do that—why now? I pleaded, I begged, I threatened, and I got you back into school. Now I'm going to have to do it again." A tear rolled out of one of Polly's eyes, and she brushed it away with the back of her hand, determined not to cry.

"They're going to expel you, Ricki," she continued in a shaky voice. "They don't have to take this, and I have no idea how I'm going to find a school that *will* take you."

Polly started the car. "Why?" she forced a steady voice. "Of all times?"

Ricki bit her lip, shrinking back in her seat, but did not answer.

Polly backed the car slowly out of the parking space. It took all her strength to control both the car and her own temper. She repeated the question, "Why?"

Ricki's eyebrows wrinkled together in concern. "I don't remember."

Polly glanced in the mirror and met her daughter's eyes for a second. Ricki's stare was a mixture of resentment and fear.

Polly's answer was half anger and half bafflement, "You don't *remember*? You have to remember; it happened less than an hour ago! Why did you do it? You *have* to have had a reason!"

"I don't know," Ricki protested, her voice shaking slightly.

Polly drew a shaky breath, trying to calm herself. "Listen to me. You kicked that kid for a reason. People don't do things like that for no reason." She turned onto the street and pointed the car toward home. "I don't know why you don't want to talk about it, but you have to, whatever the reason. I'm not going to say I won't be mad at you when you tell me, but it will be much better if you tell me now. Why did you attack that kid?"

Ricki's face puckered, and tears gathered in her brown eyes. "I don't *know* why. I remember it happened but I don't remember what I was thinking. It just happened. That's all I know."

"*Stop lying to me!*" Polly yelled. "Things like that don't 'just happen'! Stop trying to act as if it's not your fault!" Swearing as her bumper almost collided with a truck, she forced her foot to ease off the gas pedal. "It didn't just happen by itself, you did it. You *have* to remember why!"

Ricki squirmed in her seat and clenched her eyes shut, but the tears escaped, sliding down her face. "I'm not lying," she whimpered, her lower jaw sticking out in defiance. "I don't remember why. *You're* lying, because you say I have to remember, and I *don't.*"

A wave of fury almost overcame Polly. She gripped the steering wheel tightly to maintain her self-control. "You don't talk to your mother that way," she said in a low, dangerous voice. "You don't call your mother a liar!"

"You called me a liar *first!*"

"That's because you weren't telling the truth, and you know it!" Rage mixed with despair now, and there were tears of frustration in Polly's eyes too. How stupid did Ricki think she was? How dense and arrogant could a child be, expecting people to believe her ridiculous story?

You're the parent, she told herself. Get a grip. She forced herself to speak calmly, "Ricki, it is simply not possible for someone to kick someone else without having a reason for it. What you have been saying to me is not believable. You must realize that and stop expecting me to believe it. Now I want you to relax, think about when you kicked that kid, and tell me what was in your mind when you did it."

Ricki slumped forward, shaking in angry sobs. "I can't," she cried. "When I think about it I don't remember anything in my mind. *I can't.*"

The car came to an abrupt stop in the driveway. "We're home," said Polly. "Go to your room and think about it until you have an answer for me. I'm going to talk to your doctor."

The phone shook in Polly's hand as she recounted the events of the day to Ricki's psychiatrist. "Ricki kept saying she didn't know why. Why did she say that? Why didn't she just tell me why she did it?" Polly demanded, struggling to keep the tears away.

When the doctor said nothing, Polly continued. "I mean, I don't understand! She's done things like this before, too, saying she doesn't know things that she must know. Partly, I'm angry at Ricki for assuming that I'm *stupid* enough to believe the stories she tells, and partly I'm concerned, because I keep feeling that she must have some terrible secret, something that I ought to know about, something she thinks she has to lie about and hide."

After a long pause, the doctor said quietly, "I think she really doesn't know."

For a moment it felt like all the world was turning against her. The last thing Polly expected was this calm confirmation of her daughter's bizarre claim.

"How can Ricki not *know*?" Polly cried. "Ricki knows how to spell almost every word in the dictionary, knows grammar better than her teachers do, knows how the exhaust system of a car works, knows every phase of the life cycle of a ladybug..."

"She doesn't know why she hurts people," the doctor said. "That's how impulses are. People don't always know why they do things, especially children, especially a child like Ricki. When she loses impulse control, it's not her conscious mind making a choice; it's her emotional handicaps making her do things she really doesn't want to do, things that scare her when she realizes what has happened."

"You mean she was telling the truth?"

"I think so."

"Oh." Polly sagged, then shuddered as the reality took hold. In all her conversations with Ricki's psychiatrist, about Ricki's emotional disorders and impulse-control problems, the idea that Ricki had no idea what was happening when her compulsions took over simply had never registered in Polly's mind. Now, as she saw things from Ricki's point of view, she felt miserable herself.

Polly imagined the classroom from a child's viewpoint: another student came near, a sudden destructive rage surged up, then the student was on the floor, clutching a bruised leg, as the girl who has bruised it trembled in fear of the monster inside her. She saw the long hallway ahead of the child being led to the principal's office, and she felt Ricki's anxiety, wondering what Mother would say.

Finally, Polly saw herself in the car moments ago, scolding as tears burned Ricki's eyes. She knew that in Ricki's mind there was no middle ground. Truth was truth, lies were lies, and when adults, even her mother, dismissed the truth as a lie, Ricki would file it as a bitter injustice and remember it for years.

"So what do I do?" Polly murmured. "Tell me, what can I do when something like that happens?"

"It's a hard question," the doctor said sympathetically. "You've been given a difficult role in this child's life. To Ricki, her parents are supposed to be a refuge from the rest of the world. The rest of the world doesn't understand her; and it teases, punishes, and rejects her, and when she comes home to you, she needs you to be there for her."

"Be there for her."

"Of course, it's still your duty to tell her what she should and shouldn't do, and to try your best to stop her from hurting people. But if she's going to grow past this stage and learn to consider other people's feelings, she has to have someone who considers *her* feelings, someone who listens to her. Ricki is a child who needs a lot of listening, a lot of attention and acceptance. Sometimes it's hard to listen and accept her when she has done things that simply cannot be accepted."

Polly nodded, pressing her lips together. "So when I tell her that her behavior is unacceptable, I have to do it gently, while letting her know that I accept *her.*"

"Yes, exactly," murmured the psychiatrist, "You have to be sure she knows you're talking about her behavior, and not about her as a person, because, of course, you accept her as a person."

"Exactly," Polly repeated.

Guilt descended on Polly like a smothering blanket. "I've done everything so wrong. I haven't accepted her. I've shouted at her, rejected her, told her she was lying, ordered her to tell me something she didn't know. And I've done things like this so many times. I've ruined her life. It's probably all my fault that she has so many problems."

"No, it isn't. This is simply how she is, how she was born. Thousands of children are born with the same problems, to all kinds of parents, good and bad. From all the time I've worked with your family, I can tell you that, as parents, you're on the good end of the scale. You do accept her, much more often than society expects you to. You encourage her when she does good, intelligent things; you answer her questions patiently and clearly; you are there for her when someone hurts her."

"I wasn't there for her today. I should have been there for her. I should have realized what was happening and what she needed, but I was stupid and failed her."

"Failure happens. Parents aren't perfect, especially when the child is as infuriating as Ricki can be. All parents lose their tempers sometimes, and a lot of the time the anger is misplaced. You acted in a way that would have been more appropriate if Ricki were a normal girl."

"But she isn't, and that's why she did what she did today. I failed her by not realizing that."

The doctor paused, then spoke with a hint of cheer behind his calm voice. "I'm sure you've heard that we all have to learn from our mistakes; that failure exists to prepare us for success later. So, learn from this mistake, and let this failure strengthen you to succeed another time. I'm not here to be *your* psychiatrist, but I can give advice to help you and your daughter deal with the problems that you both face. Here's a bit of that advice: When you think about a problem you've had, don't think only of what you did wrong. Consider what the experience has taught you, and know that, because of it, things will be better next time."

Polly hung up the phone with hands that were steadier than before, although they still shook slightly. She walked down the hall to her daughter's room and knocked quietly.

There was no answer.

Opening the door a crack, and looking in, she saw the aftermath of a tantrum. Pillows and blankets had been flung around the room, a doll and a toy car had been smashed, there was a new dent in the plaster wall, and several childish drawings that had hung on Ricki's magnet board lay shredded on the floor.

In the midst of it, Ricki slept sprawled across her bed, her face flushed and tearstained.

Polly shut the door. The next time she would talk to Ricki quietly. Walking away from Riki's door, her whisper was more of a prayer for the strength she would need than a statement:

"A little bit better next time."

Love Letter

The letter was sprawled over my desk, an entire sheet of paper with words scribbled across it in pencil. Only a few words; the bare minimum for such a letter. "I love you." And then a signature: "José."

I barely knew José. I wasn't the type who made friends with everyone in my grade school classes. Certainly José had never paid attention to me. I could recognize him: a muscular boy of medium height, with nut-brown skin and a Mexican accent. His thick black hair looked oiled, and was always carefully combed and arranged. But I knew nothing about his personality.

Was he secretly attracted to me? The idea made me tremble with excitement. Love was mysterious and fascinating; I read love stories with a sort of wonder. The physical expressions of love meant little to me at the time, but I daydreamed of being cherished, of someone calling me beautiful. It could be José.

Or, far more likely, it could be a joke, as it had been half a dozen times before. But I didn't want to believe that.

"Look," I announced. "Do you suppose this is really from José?"

"Let me see," said Becky. "No, I think this is fake, Erika. What jerks. Just ignore it."

I must have looked crestfallen. "Don't worry about it," said Becky, patting my shoulder. "They think it's funny to play jokes on you, but it isn't. They're just stupid immature boys. They see that you're a little bit different, and that's all they notice; they don't see that you're a person. They don't realize how great you are. But someday there'll be a guy who does."

I sighed, going back to my desk. Reason told me Becky was right. If José loved me, why tell me so in a scribbled note of three words, and why leave it lying wide open across my desk for everyone to see, instead of folding it carefully and putting my name on it?

But emotion was obstinate. I wanted someone to be in love with me. What if the note was real and I ignored it? I would be hurting José; I would be losing my own chance for love. I couldn't risk that. I had to get other opinions.

"I got this letter. Who do you think wrote it?"
"Probably some annoying kid wanting to make a fool out of you. Throw it away."

"Look at this note. Do you think José left it on my desk?"
"You are so dumb. I can't believe you can't tell that's fake."

"I found this. It's not from José, is it?"
A smirk, a concealed chuckle. "Well, that sure looks like José's handwriting. I think it is."

When school let out, I almost danced downstairs to my afterschool latchkey program, the paper folded and clasped in my hand. It was José's handwriting. José was in love with me. It didn't matter now that people teased me about my clothes and my social ineptitude. I had found someone who loved me.

At latchkey, the teachers brought out a box full of all different things. Yarn and beans and beads and Popsicle sticks and chenille sticks and glitter and glue and bits of fabric and walnut shells. "Go ahead and make whatever you like."

During the past week, I had been creating a family of baby snakes. I made them out of pipe cleaners, tied tiny ribbons around their necks, built them beds and strollers and playhouses and toys of their own. It was my great project of that year of latchkey, and I had a complete snake nursery with all the necessities and entertainments that a baby snake could possibly want.

But that day I abandoned the project. Instead of a new piece of snake paraphernalia, I made a tiny box. I took two walnut shells, made a hinge of masking tape and a clasp and four tiny curled feet out of pipe cleaners, and then set about decorating the top. Dozens of bits of black yarn, glued thickly together for hair. Red yarn for a mouth. Black arches of yarn for eyebrows. Beans and beads were not satisfactory for the beautiful eyes I wanted to make, so I drew them on with marker, then made two smaller marks for a nose.

"Who's that?"

"My boyfriend," I said dreamily.

In those days I couldn't sleep without listening to music. I had a tape that I played every night. Lying curled up in my blanket, I smiled at the words of an old song. The musician seemed to speak of my life, singing that everyone would someday know the experience of loving and being loved.

Everybody loved somebody at some time, and my time had come. I had never truly been in love before, I had never before won anyone's heart. But now I was finally somebody.

Back at school, I saw José with new eyes. I looked for love in every one of his movements, imagined that he watched me every time I turned my eyes away. Soon, I told myself, we would sit together all the time, we would walk down the halls holding hands. For now, it was enough to know that he loved me.

Or perhaps it wasn't. Because I was impatient; I wanted to feel what it was like to talk with someone who loved me, I wanted to learn to whisper endearments and flattery the way people did in books. I wanted to be together. But I didn't know how to begin.

It was a break in class. I had been watching him from afar for hours, when two other boys walked up to me.

"José really likes you," one of them said.

"Yes, he does," I murmured happily.

"Why don't you go kiss him?" said the other, grinning.

Why not? If José loved me, he wouldn't object. I didn't know any other way of letting him know that I accepted his love. I got up and walked toward him.

The two boys leaned together, watching. A crowd of other kids solidified around them, breath held, eyes on me.

I walked forward. José was leaning over the bookshelf, putting a book back in place. His head was tilted down; he didn't see me.

Closer. Close enough to touch him. I took a breath. I leaned my hand on the bookshelf.

And then, all at once, I put my arms around him and kissed him. I wasn't in a good position to direct the kiss; it landed on the side of his head, almost his neck.

A second later I was pushed back. "What the hell? What are you doing? Get away from me!" José threw me off and backed into the wall, wiping at his face. "Geez!"

The crowd of boys burst out laughing. "Good going, Erika!" one of them yelled. Blushing in shame, I returned to my desk and buried my head in my arms.

I wish I could say that I tore up the note and threw it away; that after being so stupid, I learned a little sense. But I didn't. My desire to believe overcame all logic. I told myself that maybe José was just shocked at being kissed so suddenly; that maybe he would still love me if I went slowly from then on.

I kept the letter for months, pinned to the bulletin board in my bedroom, just in case it might somehow be real.

Prairie Dog

When I was in fourth grade, I had been to North and South Dakota with my parents, and had seen colonies of prairie dogs. They were charming creatures: like squirrels, but brown and short-tailed, living in elaborate underground complexes. In some places they were so tame that tourists could crouch by their burrows and feed them peanuts when they came up.

My parents bought me a sweatshirt with a picture of a family of prairie dogs on it. It could have been a picture from a nature encyclopedia—a drawing, but realistic to the last detail, with a bit of grass and soil in the foreground. In the corner, in small type, were the words "Prairie Dog."

I wore it to school. I liked it; the prairie dogs were cute, and it was a comfortable shirt. I didn't think about it much; I never thought much about my daily clothes ... unless they caused an unforeseen problem. In the case of this shirt, the problem was something neither I nor my parents could ever have predicted.

I was sitting at my desk, doodling on my folder and waiting for class to start, when a boy walked past my seat in the classroom. He fixed his eyes on me, smirked, and called out "Prairie dog!"

Bizarre, idiotic, and yet I could tell it was meant to hurt me. For me, where there was the intent to offend, there was offense.

Anger burst up, impossible to suppress. I looked up and scowled at him, and he ran away, laughing.

When class was over, we lined up to go into the next room for math class. As I found my place in line, a girl brushed close by me, whispering in my ear, "Prairie dog!"

Angry heat stabbed through me again, a reflex I couldn't control. I swung around and lunged at her, wanting to hit but not actually intending to, meaning only to scare her away. It worked. She giggled madly and dashed off to the other end of the room, where she called again, "Prairie dog!" before taking her own place in line.

At lunch, children at another table watched me eat, crying out, "Prairie dog!" every few seconds, and then pretending not to notice me when I looked up at them. By the end of the meal I was tense, my teeth were bared, my nerves were on edge.

I spent recess as far from the other students as I could, but they would run past me and shout, "Prairie dog!" If I ran after them, they eluded me, hid behind an aide, and then came back to yell, "Prairie dog!" again as soon as they thought it might be safe.

Halfway through recess, angry and hurt, I went to the aide. "Everyone teases me about my shirt," I complained. "They yell 'Prairie dog!' at me."

"Ignore them. They'll stop," was the simple answer, and I could get no other.

I couldn't ignore them, and they didn't stop.

The next few days I didn't even wear the shirt, but the remarks surged up again. When I came into the classroom in the morning, the first thing I heard was, "Prairie dog!"

It became a regular sport. Variations developed. "Hey, look, there's a prairie dog!" someone would call, pointing energetically. When I turned in that direction without thinking, everyone would burst out laughing and yell, "Made you look!"

I learned to look in the opposite direction. That didn't stop them. They would simply change the direction they were pointing. "Prairie dog! Made you look!"

I kept my face buried in my hands. "Prairie dog in your hand! Made you look!"

I closed my eyes. "Prairie dog inside your eyelids! Made you look!"

Were they deliberately playing on how sensitive I was to teasing? Did they know how badly it wounded me, how difficult it was for me to control my reactions? Did they know how close I was to crying, how close to attacking somebody? Was that the reason they continued to torment me?

It was a break in class. I sat in a corner, hiding my face in a book, praying that no one would make fun of me again. I was going crazy. If it happened one more time ...

"Prairie dog!"

Seconds later, a classmate was crouched on the floor clutching his face in pain, and my hand stung from the impact.

"Why did you hit him?" asked the principal's aide, her arms folded across her chest.

"He teased me about my shirt. Everybody teased me about my shirt. They yelled, 'Prairie dog!' I couldn't stand it anymore."

"What had you said about your shirt?"

"I didn't say anything about it. I just wore it, once."

"That can't be true. You must have made some big deal about it. You must have egged them on to tease you somehow. People don't tease you unless you make a big deal. Nobody gets teased if they don't want to."

I sank into pure rage, because the only thing that could make me angrier than teasing was somebody believing a lie, and the worst kind of lie was a false accusation.

What did she mean? I wondered, riding home on the bus. Did normal people want to be teased? Did they encourage their friends to make fun of them? Did they find real enjoyment in what was excruciating pain to me?

And if they did, why was it assumed that I did the same? While some people judged me entirely on their stereotypes of children with mental disabilities, other people took it for granted that I felt everything normal children felt.

Would people ever understand me?

Virgin

Dinner with my friends had gone badly that night. Alone, wishing I could sleep, I wondered why I still made any social efforts at all. Why did I go out to eat with people when I knew I would just make an idiot of myself? Why did I let myself be lured into an evening out by the promise that a nice guy would be there, someone I'd had a crush on? I had to know that it would end the way it always did.

I was lying in bed, alone, lonely, angry at the world for shutting me out and forcing me to be alone. Angry at myself for being such a misfit in the world that it had to shut me out.

Mostly, angry that nobody desired me, that I probably wouldn't ever have any chance of losing my virginity, that I didn't know how to dress to attract men, even how to talk to attract them. Angry at myself because whenever I found a guy attractive, I went up to him and made crude jokes about wanting to tear off his clothes, and as a result he neither felt comfortable with me nor took my desire seriously. From that moment on, I was just a freak to him, not even a person. Why did I let it happen again and again?

I should have expected that, when I finally fell asleep that night, some miserable outcast would intrude on my dreams.

Another Friday night spent alone in his room.

No one to take to a hotel for the weekend, no one with whom to work out his bottled-up passions for a night in his own bedroom. Not even a bedroom of his own—he didn't have to share his bedroom, but it didn't belong to him; he didn't own it. He was undoubtedly the only student in the whole college who still lived with his mother.

He admitted that he was hard to get along with. Hard enough that no place of employment had ever kept him longer than a few weeks. Hard enough that he had no established group of friends to go out with on lonely nights like this. So hard, in fact, that at the age of 24 he was still a virgin.

Was there some meaning to all this?

He had always suspected that the universe planned something out of the ordinary for his life. All the great historical figures had been ignored, ostracized, sometimes punished by their contemporaries before they proved themselves worthy. At first the world saw only someone who was different, and shied away, but later it learned who he was, and the greatness he offered. The stone the builders rejected became the cornerstone. Had Christ ever married?

His mother knocked on the door to the bedroom that was not his.

"Are you working on your paper?"

"No." A short, resentful answer.

"Is something wrong?" She opened the door.

He sighed, thinking that people who intruded deserved any shocks they got. "To tell you the blatant truth, I happen to be upset because I'm almost a quarter of a century old and no one has ever offered to have sex with me."

"Oh?"

"Yeah."

"Well, think of all the worries you're escaping. No venereal diseases, no paternity suits. And plenty of time to work on your sociology paper."

"Shut up! I doubt Mary was ever this cruel to Jesus."

"Oh, there you go again. You had better be careful of those delusions of grandeur, you know. All the great tyrants of history had them. What do you want me to do? Hire you a prostitute?"

"Actually, I want you to go away."

"Oh, why didn't you say so? I'd be honored." The door started to close.

"Wait."

"What now?"

"You *can* do something for me. Tell me about my childhood."

"What about it?"

"Anything. Did anything ever happen when I was young that made you think I might do something worthwhile with my life?"

"Like save the world from sin?"

"You don't have to make that assumption, Mom! That is not necessarily what I mean. I'm open to a lot of possibilities! Maybe be a president, or a famous activist, or even just a successful person at all?"

"Well, you were born to a virgin."

"Shut up, Mom. I mean seriously."

"Seriously, yes. This is something I have been meaning to tell you for years. This happened to be the week I promised myself I would get around to it, and when you asked me that question, I thought, this must be the moment."

"What the hell do you mean?"

"Have you ever seen your father? Have I ever told you who he was? That's the reason. I was a virgin when you were born, and I'm still a virgin now, and therefore you were the product of a virgin birth. So take that and let your messiah complex make what it likes of it."

He sat down heavily on his bed. Even though his mother had managed to keep some things from him all his life, he had learned to tell when she was serious. And now, out of nowhere, she had given him a hope that, despite his fantasies of greatness, he had never been able to take quite seriously.

The feeling had been there. The sense that greatness was calling him, that he was destined to change the world, and now he knew that the feeling wasn't a mistake, only an understatement.

This revelation of his birth opened him to hopes higher than any he had considered in any depth. Presidents weren't born of virgins. Neither were activists or successful businessmen.

Questions struggled to be asked. Why did it take you so long to tell me this? And then, You always laughed at my hopes. Why did you tell me at all? Then, the hostility draining from him, and an awed gentleness replacing it, he said, "Did any angels come to you in a dream?"

"I don't remember angels. I had some weird dreams during the pregnancy. Once I dreamt I was a slug."

He winced. "Did you ever hear a voice from heaven telling you that you were chosen to bear a holy child? Did a beam of light surround you as I came into the world?"

"Of course not. Why are you acting as if this were something supernatural?"

"Because what else could it be?" he demanded, his voice rising nearly to a shout. "You just told me that you gave birth to me without having sex. Haven't you ever wondered how it happened?"

"Why would I? They explained it all very clearly."

"Who did?"

"The people at the sperm bank."

There was a pause that crashed the way a tsunami crashes after seeming to rise to the sky and beyond.

"You were fertilized at a sperm bank?"

"Of course."

"Even though you were a virgin?"

"Of course."

"Why?"

"I wanted a baby."

"But why didn't you try the normal way first?"

"Because no one would have sex with me," she said, turning to leave. "I thought telling you that would make you feel better."

I woke up laughing. Then, as I thought about the meaning of the dream, I felt more like crying, because however lonely and virginal he was, the sullen young man with the delusions of godhood didn't represent me.

I was the mother.

In My Own World

It's not surprising that many people with Asperger's Syndrome feel like aliens. An autistic life is like being on an alien planet, researching the customs of a different species, lacking the social instincts that the natives possess and trying to figure out what to expect through reason instead of intuition.

Sometimes, our only relief is inventing cultures of our own that make more sense to us. Throughout my struggle, that's how I have kept myself entertained, satisfied my need for a world I could fit into, and gradually learned enough about cultures that I could understand the one I was born into.

Before I learned some of the customs of the human species, I was, indeed, an alien on my own planet. I didn't understand the actions of my fellow humans and I found them stupid and meaningless, and yet I wanted very much to fit in. I wanted to have friends. I wanted to be accepted as I was, instead of being rejected because I was different. I wanted to be loved.

Even in third and fourth grade I daydreamed all the time about being in love, but my attempts to win romantic affection were always inappropriate, and resulted only in laughter and ridicule. The boys I pursued were never attracted to me in the first place; mostly their love was professed by fun-seeking third parties. I couldn't pick up the social clues that would have told me it was a trick.

By the time I was thirteen our home was full of my "books," stapled-together sheets of paper on which I had written tales of fantasy and science fiction, of humor and adventure, of children in grade school, and of people who traveled to magical secret worlds or met alien creatures. The more familiar I became with science fiction, the more my ideas leaned in that direction.

I began to believe that, like a man who feels he should have been a woman, I had been put in the wrong body, except that in my case the mistake was interplanetary. I had been born in a world I couldn't understand, a world where students who studied were laughed at, a world where people could get genuinely angry about the color of a dress or a living room, a world where more money was put into football than education or feeding the hungry. I couldn't fit into this world, so I felt the need to create a world of my own.

At that time, like many thirteen-year-olds, I rebelled against the power that adults have over children. I created the *Erilcans*, a humanoid species whose culture reversed the age roles in society. A young Erilcan gained all the rights and responsibilities of a human adult as soon as he declared himself ready for them, and then lost them when he turned 18, whereupon he was put in a government-funded home until he had children who were ready to support him.

By making Erilcans physically and mentally almost identical to humans, I implied that such a system would work with the human species. Although ridiculous, it was a powerful expression of my own outrage as a precocious teenager. I knew I was intelligent. Despite my youth, I was perceptive enough to see how stupidly adults could act sometimes, yet I had to obey them by virtue of our ages alone.

I filled notebook after notebook with information on the Erilcans — their legal system, the foods they ate, the other life forms on their planet, the geography of their world and their solar system, even an Erilcan Constitution. I wrote a play and a book about them, and I made some of their clothing and artifacts for myself. I made up their language.

It was wonderful. I had a world I fit into! On Erilca the rulers were all teenage girls. On Erilca, culture was based on the enjoyment of life. The Erilcan psyche was a lot like mine at the time: energetic, funny, exuberant, with almost annoyingly high self-esteem even in the face of hatred. On Erilca, I would be normal.

As I grew older, the world I fit into became different, so I made new ones. After the Erilcans came the *Andromedians*, a shape-changing species who lived on Andromedia II, the second inhabited planet to be discovered in the Galaxy Andromeda. I wrote a screenplay and a novel about them, too, and filled half of a thick green journal with their culture.

Andromedians were made of a claylike, flexible mass controlled by an unchanging brain. They married by physically joining with each other. A joined couple could have a child by "morphing" a part of itself into a brain, with all the necessary physical parts to learn, process information, and control a body. Then that brain, attached to enough flesh to form the rest of its body parts, would be cut off and learn to live on its own.

Once born, Andromedians could stretch and sculpt their bodies to take on any physical form they wished. Many chose to resemble humans or other Earth creatures, but no one was condemned for creating a shape completely from imagination.

The Andromedians had been studying Earth through interplanetary probes since 500 BC, and had based their culture on human cultures, adding many beliefs unique to them and me. For example, they couldn't see the point of dinner conversation. (Why should two actions that involve the same part of the body take place simultaneously? If talking with one's mouth full is impolite, why use mealtimes as the main talking events of the day?)

Gender was merely a custom borrowed from humans, and one could decide whether to be male, female, both, or neither. Appearance was entirely up to the individual. There were fashions, but they did not rule one's existence; creativity was encouraged in those areas, and in all areas of life.

Andromedian brains were particularly suited to storing information that made sense. Trying to live by pointless Earth customs had resulted in insanity where both the perception of what made sense and the perception of what was accepted by custom went wildly awry. Each Andromedian began to experience occasional lapses early in adolescence; these, of course, were the Andromedian version of my own attacks of hyperactive behavior, described as physical events as common as menstruation.

Strange though these fantasies might seem, they helped. Through years of studying and learning by experience, I began to understand this complicated place called Earth. Creating other worlds helped me live in this one. I realized humanity was a culture I had to learn. I explored its idiosyncrasies by imagining different ones, and slowly that helped me begin to fit in.

At times I still have difficulty keeping track of the illogical customs of this planet. I still find myself offending people without meaning to; sometimes I still don't know if I'm saying the right thing until I see people's reactions, and sometimes I misinterpret those. I still have trouble remembering names; I still get hyperactive sometimes; I still often feel safer being alone.

Yet I have become an Earthling in most of my visible aspects. I have a better idea of how to dress; I have made considerable progress in the art of conversation; my episodes of silliness are less frequent. I can manage a small home by myself; I know how to use public transportation; I can register for classes on my own. I have friends who respect me and even think I am brilliant.

I continue to create planets, but the species I invent are less like me. Creating them has become a pastime in which I indulge just for fun. My latest inventions do not symbolize my life; they merely reflect my growing interest in culture, language, and people. Having learned so much about cultures, I find them turning into a hobby.

After I worked on the Andromedians for some time, I painted several pictures of a third species called *Springers*. The Springers also lived on Andromedia II. According to the paintings, they hunted while riding on domesticated flying predators, bathed by sitting in a pool and allowing pet fish to eat the dirt off them, ate fruits that grew on the tentacles of a tame creature called the Wheelberry Beast, and played a sport like life-sized chess. They had armlike tentacles and three spring-shaped legs, and came in three sexes and at least two races, which differed in the number of arms and the way they ate.

After I met my best friend, who also created alien worlds, I came up with yet another: the parallel humans, who lived on Earth in an alternate universe. They had never developed conquest; the borders of the countries remained the same for thousands of years. I filled the other half of the green journal with the history of that Earth, especially ancient Greece, whose traditions and religion had barely changed since 3000 BC, despite advances in technology. I created a language and some of the culture (for example, on parallel Earth the most common animal to be bred as a pet is not the dog or cat, but the parrot).

My latest is the world of the *Circle People*, who communicate using a "Speaking Circle," a special tool made up of a disc and 27 tiny carved shapes that can be arranged on the disc in different patterns, each of which represents a word. I have made my own Speaking Circle and I'm working on the language. People admire it and say I'm creative.

As I have become more familiar with the culture I live in—the human culture—creating new worlds has stopped being a way to escape from the "real" world and make myself a place to fit in. It's now just a way to have fun and impress my friends. But when I first knew the feeling that I had been born on the wrong planet, creating other worlds was a means of survival.

Beautiful

I knew I looked beautiful. I had seen beauty in the mirror that morning when I had stood back to admire my clothes, my jewelry, my makeup. I could tell beauty when I saw it, and I looked beautiful.

I was wearing a flowing orange skirt with a gentle ruffle around the bottom, and yellow and red flowers twining intricately across the fabric. Also a dark red, skin-tight tank top, of a soft unpatterned cloth—the only decorations were the faintly shiny bands of the collar and cuffs. Someone had said red didn't go with orange. Ridiculous. Look at the top of a rainbow. Nature thought they went together; I wasn't going to argue with that.

The skirt came to just above my ankles. If people looked closely, they would see that I didn't shave my legs, but the shoes would probably distract them from that: hot-pink suede, shaped like cowboy boots but coming up only to a few inches below the hem of my skirt. They had slits in the sides with elastic in them, to slip easily onto my feet.

I wore no bra under the red top, because the wide neck would show bra straps. The neck had to be wide enough to allow for my necklace, an elaborate collar of clear rhinestones and silver filigree that might have been found on a European empress of ages past. I had bought it amazingly cheap at an antique store down the street from my house. It was big enough to cover any scabs from the pimples I'd squeezed on my chest. I wouldn't wear anything smaller with a shirt this low-necked.

Pine-green, iridescent glass beads hung from my ears; I wore a gilded tennis bracelet of pink and clear rhinestones; my fingers were encircled in rings of all possible kinds. There was a square garnet on an undulating silver band, bought at a store that also sold crystals with magical healing powers. There was my prized piece of amber with a tiny mosquito in it, which I'd had put in a setting so elegant it could have been an engagement ring. There were the antique ruby and emerald rings that my grandmother had given me, the gold-plating wearing off their ancient bands.

I had carefully outlined my mouth and then covered it thickly in very dark lipstick. It was "Fawn Fatale," the color that made my mom comment, with a snort, that it made me look like a dead deer. A heavy dusting of pink brought out each of my cheekbones. My eyebrows were slender brown arches, and the spaces between them and my eyes were full of purple and glitter. My fingernails were metallic gold covered with a layer of transparent blue.

I'd braided my hair on each side, and coiled it into buns held in place by the combined effort of dozens of bobby pins. In one braid I stuck a pin bejeweled with faceted glass, something my mother was given when she was my age and then gave to me. All over both sides of my hair were little flowers made of iridescent pastel plastic, each bearing a small rhinestone. They had been a gift from my cousin, and they attached to my hair with Velcro.

As I walked down the stairs, I caught another glimpse of myself in the hallway mirror. Beautiful. Nobody would be able to look away from me. I paused, long enough to give my reflection a seductive smile, and went to catch the bus to school.

Making up My Mind

The first time I put on makeup I was about 12. I wanted to make myself unrecognizable and see if people recognized me anyway, having been inspired by a curly red wig I had found among my mom's old things. All masters of disguise do something to alter their faces, and since my mom possessed nothing more daring than strawberry Chapstick, it was necessary for me to go off on a makeup quest.

I was a regular customer at Butler Drug, my chosen source of makeup, but most of the merchandise that had passed into my hands there had been SweeTARTS and Laffy Taffy. I felt a little nervous buying the tube of cherry-red lipstick and the pink rouge, as if someone might ask me to produce an ID card and prove myself competent to choose cosmetics. No one did, and my heart slowed to a regular beat as I walked down to my favorite bookstore to unleash my plan upon the unsuspecting world.

My plan was to astonish the cashiers. None of them knew what I had in my bag until I slipped into the little bathroom and emerged dramatically with curly red hair, a crimson mouth, and surreally blushing cheeks. The result was a torrent of laughter and applause behind the counter, followed by an equal torrent of constructive criticism concerning my makeup.

My version of the adolescent cosmetic craze had begun. It continued for four years. Those were the years when I kept lipstick in my belt-pack; when I put on nail polish in class; when I threw away whole ten-dollar bills on lip colors that some people wouldn't have been able to distinguish from shades I already owned. I consider myself wholly unique and cringe at describing my actions with the word "normal," but for four years I was the stereotypical teen whose cheeks aren't red enough, whose lips aren't well enough defined, and who won't feel secure with herself until foreign bodies are adhered to her face to imitate natural beauty.

It wasn't normal in all ways, though. It ended. I don't wear makeup any more. Not because I realized in a blinding flash that makeup was stupid and pointless. I'd known that already. I'd known it was demeaning. I'd known it was an insult to my real face. I'd known that its only purpose was to attract men, and that even if it succeeded, they wouldn't be the kind of men I would want to be with.

I had known that billions of dollars are spent on producing makeup, buying makeup, and using the media to convince more people to buy it. Money that could save hundreds of millions of lives, if put to other uses, is constantly poured into making women feel insecure and unsatisfactory, as if they were broken and had to be stuck back together with mascara and nail polish. I had known perfectly well that by buying makeup I was proving that I suffered from one of the flaws for which I most pitied normal people: the capacity to fall for that sort of moneymaking scheme.

I wore makeup anyway.

Gradually lipstick and blush lost their allure. I noticed the hours I struggled to catch up, having spent my class time worrying about my nails; the dozens of dollars I was spending on artificial beauty while claiming not to care how I looked. I realized that what I really wanted was not a perfect complexion, but the ability to take off my face and body and draw attention to the parts of me that I want to be judged.

Makeup is an enormous industry for the simple reason that it can make enormous amounts of money. If people can be convinced that they're not doing what they should; that is, what everyone else is doing, they will pay any price to remedy the shortcoming. Companies have played on this assumption, and become ridiculously successful. The industry has even succeeded in affecting our culture: where makeup once was considered scandalous, now it's scandalous to go without it.

Most women in this society would need great courage to break the tradition of wearing makeup. One of normal people's greatest fears is being considered abnormal in the smallest way. Fear fuels the advertising industry, and it makes manufacturers rich, but fear also breaks people into cliques and leaves naturally unusual people rejected and lonely.

Realizing the connection between makeup and the persecution I experienced all through school, I overcame my own fear of going unpainted. I acknowledge that, logically, that decision may bring less respect from some women, and less attention from some men, but what gain would makeup bring? Respect from people who base respect on appearance? Desire from people who choose an object of desire for how she looks? Superficial acceptance by people who wouldn't look beyond the paint on my skin to see me?

When people reject me, it's because they see something unsettlingly strange in my behavior, such as the way I talk, the social nuances I miss, my hyperactivity, my tics. They turn away before they have a chance to know the person as well as the disabilities. Any acceptance I could get from wearing makeup would be as shallow; people might accept my cosmetized exterior, but they wouldn't look any closer.

I know now that I would rather dress as an alien than wear makeup. A cosmetically painted face is an alien form in itself, but a costume with green tentacles would be more honest. Then, at least, I would be saying something about my personality to all who saw me. I would announce that I have a sense of humor, that I like science fiction, that I am eccentric and different from other people.

If I wore makeup, it would show that I placed a great value on physical appearance and conformity, and that would be a lie. If I wore makeup, people might make false assumptions about me; makeup would draw them away from actually getting to know me; substitute a misunderstanding for true recognition. People misunderstand me enough already!

Makeup taught me that I don't want to make myself unrecognizable to see if people recognize me anyway.

They might not.

Life of a Ladybug

"I don't like bugs," my cousin said, her five-year-old features wrinkling in anxiety at the potato beetle trundling around her feet. "Bugs are yucky. They scare me!"

I couldn't resist pointing to the six-legged red circle embroidered on her T-shirt. "Don't you like ladybugs?"

In an instant her face relaxed, and she smiled. "I don't like bugs," she amended, "except ladybugs."

Except ladybugs. We're most ready to romanticize the animals we know least about. If my cousin were more familiar with their daily lives, would she find ladybugs as lovable? I doubt it. They are born ugly, they can be merciless killers, they don't show unconditional love for their fellow ladybugs, and they die disgusting deaths.

In short, they're real. Like us, they are imperfect inhabitants of this imperfect universe, and not the fairy tale creatures that people believe them to be.

Many children with Asperger's syndrome develop strange but amazingly detailed interests. Some are able to identify any model of washing machine ever made; some know hundreds of palindromes; some can remember the date and location of every battle of the Second World War.

My fascination was ladybugs. I amassed a world of knowledge of their biology and behavior, and in studying them I found that they have many traits also found in humans, though few are traits that humans idealize. They range from the normal and sadly necessary cruelty of killing other species for food to an almost autistic disinterest in others of the same species.

Ladybugs are vicious. My mother taught me that when I was very young. Her love for them was understandable, because she was a gardener in nearly all her spare time, and ladybugs are the aphid's primary natural enemy. One of the first things I learned about ladybugs was that if I found one, I should bring it to the garden or the solarium. In my mother's opinion, if there were a ladybug on her premises, it should be someplace where it could kill and eat those tiny green vampires of floral lifeblood.

Nature seems biased in favor of garden pests, and the reproductive rate of aphids has a listing in the Guinness Book of World Records. The ladybug controls their soaring populations. I've seen aphids clustered on a plant happily sucking up its juices, massacred in minutes by a spotted Godzilla. A ladybug's mandibles are tiny but efficient, ripping apart and devouring prey.

Mom showed me ladybug eggs: elliptical towers a millimeter tall, yellow and translucent, clinging to whatever surface the mother chose. We used to catch the larvae. I found that they aren't grubs like most baby beetles, but lively predators, already hunting and killing. They have six legs, and in the middle a narrow black body with blunt head and pointed tail, almost wormlike but much shorter than a worm, banded with a few stripes of orange near the head. When the right time comes, the larva seals its tail to the closest available surface, curls up, and lets its skin become a shell to protect its metamorphosis. I saw it all happen in glass jars; I was the kind of child who made a pet of every animal I found.

Even pupating a ladybug can fend for itself. The first time I touched one of those tiny cocoons it caught my attention by rearing up on its tail for a moment. The blind reflex frightened me, as it must have frightened away many animals that tried to eat ladybugs in that vulnerable phase. Even knowing all the stages of an insect's lifecycle, I had taken some things for granted: larvae and adults move; eggs and pupae do not.

The ladybug surprised me again when it emerged. Instead of the colors that humans most often associate with its species, it was the same pale yellow as the eggs. The red and the spots came slowly in the hours afterwards, developing like a Polaroid photo.

It was the birth, childhood, and transformation of the ladybug that fascinated me, and I suppose that made sense. I was a growing child myself, and few people of any age pay much attention to ladybug deaths. It wasn't until much later, in college, that I thought about them at all.

On a group retreat in Wisconsin, staying in a cabin, I started seeing ladybugs everywhere. I knew that they find warm places and congregate together in the winter—they do it in my dorm building, after all—but I hadn't expected to spend a weekend stepping around them and picking them out of food.

They were aged, darkened to reddish-brown, dead or dying or with a death wish. Perhaps some were healthy enough to survive until spring, if they learned to avoid the hazards of indoor life. I saw one land on top of the stove-shaped fireplace and slowly stretch out its spotted shells and the wings underneath as the heat killed it. I watched them swirling around the light bulbs like moths, although they looked more like wasps when in flight, and battering themselves on the glass in the same hopeless way.

Do ladybugs really die so nonchalantly? Maybe it was just the bias of seeing a tiny event from a giant's point of view, of being accustomed to noisy deaths, and seeing something strange in a quiet one. The delicate lumbering unique to beetles is always the same to the eye of the human observer. A happy aphid-hunter walks with the same gait as a crawling silhouette imprisoned on the inside of a spherical light fixture.

While the group sat talking by candlelight on Saturday evening, there was a point when all thoughts but one disappeared from my awareness. I had noticed a ladybug stuck headfirst in the molten wax of one candle, wings and wing-covers spread and releasing endless tiny bubbles from the slowly boiling body. The lighted wick seemed to have been designed to illuminate the scene for maximum horror. The ladybug lay still and unstruggling.

In life, it never occurs to ladybugs to value each other as individuals. One only has to watch them together to know this. They simply don't interact. Except when mating, they are no more aware of one another than they are of dust and pebbles. I've seen their yellow eggs packed closely together, little patches of security for the continued abundance of the ladybug species. The mothers lay the eggs, and then leave and forget all about them.

Reassured on some instinctual level that there are plenty to take its place, and having no loved ones to mourn its passing, the ladybug gives itself up carelessly, without concern. It takes a far more complicated creature to call life holy and precious. The ladybug accepts the experiences of being born, giving birth, killing, and dying, all with perfect and sometimes frightening objectivity.

"I don't like bugs, except ladybugs." What is our conception of nature when a striped beetle subsisting quietly on potatoes seems more frightening than a ferocious predator clad in black-speckled red? Such is human nature, glorifying the creatures that are useful to us and demonizing those that harm us. But the ladybug isn't glorious, and it isn't a demon. It's just an animal, no more clean, wise, refined, gentle or innocent than any other.

Like the ladybug, many people put little value on the lives of species other than our own. In fact, many fear and degrade not only other species, but also those of our own species who look different, think differently, or come from other places. It's a normal instinct, to distrust the unknown, but I have difficulty understanding why some carry it to such lengths.

On the other hand, normal people have difficulty understanding me as well. Like the ladybug, I enjoy being alone, and I do not always show emotion where others would expect it. All of us, from the most autistic to the most average, have ladybug characteristics. But we are not dainty little polka-dotted pixies that flit around spreading love and kindness to the rest of the world.

Neither are ladybugs. Thinking of them that way is a misunderstanding. It's like thinking all women are docile little housewives. It's like thinking all children lack intelligence and responsibility. It's like thinking that people with mental and emotional disorders are all the same, needing to be watched carefully, disciplined strongly, talked to like babies. It is a stupidly simple definition of reality.

There is good and bad in all of us, and one should not make judgments until one has observed. That is reality!

Subways and Social Skills

Why do I like riding in subways and streetcars so much? Perhaps it's the novelty; those modes of transportation don't exist in Minneapolis, where I live, and I get to use them only when I visit Europe or the East Coast. But I enjoy Minneapolis's buses almost as much.

In any case, it's strange. Social skills have always been difficult for me, and on public transportation there are so many little social traps to fall into.

Almost the worst thing in any crowd is the question of looking. When my mind wanders, my eyes stand still, usually turned in whatever direction, in my position, it is most comfortable to look. And then I come out of my reverie to find that I have been staring at an old lady and she has turned her own eyes back on me reproachfully. So I turn hastily away, shift my body to a different position, and look straight ahead, where I encounter the face of the gentleman sitting across from me, who throws me a quizzical glance at my sudden focus on him, driving my gaze out the window.

But then I start to become uncomfortable from the glare of the sun, or we go into a tunnel and I am suddenly watching a dark featureless wall go by, which doesn't look like a normal thing to watch, and before people can begin to stare at me, I must find a new focus. The ceiling? The floor? Neither is comfortable for my neck and neither would seem natural to the observer, but the floor is slightly better on both counts. Luckily the man across from me has left by now, taking his feet with him, and my eyes have a few empty inches to rest on.

Two ladies come and sit down where he was. I am looking at feet again. Meanwhile I have let my concentration lapse a moment, and my head is again drifting to the most comfortable position for how I am now seated—neck bent slightly, eyes in the centers of their orbits—and I end up staring into the lap of the woman opposite me. As soon as I realize it, I hurry and turn to look at my reflection in the other window ... which is only a few degrees away from looking at the old lady, and she, not seeing the difference, glares at me again. And so my eyes are off once more on their endless journey, trying to find a place to rest.

And then there is always the seating problem. Should I sit in a single seat or a double seat? If I sit in a single seat, will an elderly or handicapped person have more expectation of me to get up? Maybe I should stand; after all, I can stand perfectly well, and that would leave a seat open for anyone who needs it more than I do.

But if I stand, will I be blocking the door or the aisle? What if I sit in a double seat? Should I pick one that already has someone sitting in one of the seats, or should I pick one that has both seats free? If I pick one that's all empty, should I sit in the window seat and risk having someone else take the aisle seat before I get out, so I will have to ask him to move? Or should I sit in the aisle seat and block an empty window seat from other people? And if I choose a double seat that's half taken, should it be one with an empty window seat or an empty aisle seat ... should I sit in an aisle seat and block the person in the window seat from leaving, or should I climb over someone in an aisle seat to get to the window seat he is blocking?

Heaven forbid that someone will come in with a crying baby. Nature has carefully designed a baby's cry to push the human mind into a state of near-panic. It's quite logical, ensuring that few children will go uncared-for, but sometimes I can't help but ask, why me? I have no babies and no plans to have them, but I still hear the cry as an alarm, profoundly distressing, far worse than a mere annoying noise. Demanding an answer, demanding some help I can't give, because the baby isn't mine, just a stranger's on the subway.

I'm doomed to listen to it helplessly, to endure all the alarms it sets off in my unwilling system, to hope against hope that the parent can somehow make it be quiet. Worse than a fire alarm, because every time I've ever heard a fire alarm, I've been 90% sure that it was either a drill or a prank. A screaming child is an alarm bred into millions of generations of human beings, impossible to ignore.

All these threats to my calm, and yet I seem to find my greatest relaxation and reflection while using public transportation. There is a certain peace in riding a bus or subway or streetcar. There's something so relaxing about the gentle motion of the wheels underneath me, the scenery going slowly by. It's a time to sit quietly and reflect, to write in a journal, to watch and listen to the people around me. I get some of my best ideas while riding.

Language Camp

Every summer from the year I was seven until the year I was 18, I went to language camp. I had learned German at the same time I learned my mother tongue of English, so it began with Waldsee, the Concordia Language Villages German camp in Bemidji, Minnesota. Later I added Spanish to my repertoire, and started going to the same organization's Spanish camps as well, in various sites. Early on I took two-week sessions, and later four-week sessions, sometimes more than one a year.

At Waldsee we learned to sing a song that contained the lines, "Deutsche Kultur, Freunde kennenlernen in der Natur." Translated: "German culture, meeting friends in nature." This was a good summary of the Concordia Language Villages camps' purpose, which combines language immersion with playing, socializing, and living in cabins in northern Minnesota's wilderness.

I loved the wilderness and the language immersion—finding bugs and toads and speaking German or Spanish all the time was my element—but just as in school, playing and socializing with the other children was a challenge.

The reasons were the usual ones for me: I didn't understand social life; I was hyperactive and behaved like a total maniac sometimes. The other kids shunned me for those reasons, afraid to interact with someone they didn't understand. I found it easier to have fun alone than to try and push through the walls they built between themselves and me.

When I did get involved in social interaction, sometimes disasters resulted. The most embarrassing, and I'm sorry to say, typical, happened when I had a cabinmate who was the daughter of a presidential candidate, though I had no idea until years later that her father was running for President. I chatted with her as I did with everyone else, awkwardly and carelessly, on what I thought were interesting topics: the thousands of tiny frogs down by the pond; a prize I had won for German-speaking; my opinion that my brother had no social skills.

One day I stumbled into the wrong subject completely. Stephanie, another girl in our cabin, had been bragging about her popularity with boys; Trina had told someone else, in my hearing, that she believed Stephanie was making it all up. I made the faux pas of quoting Trina's statement in Stephanie's hearing. Trina found out that I had done this, approached me and said, "You know how you're always saying your brother has no social skills? Well, you're no better, because you have absolutely none."

This made for plenty of entertainment in the years since then: I have great fun telling people that the daughter of a presidential candidate once accused me of having no social skills, but at the time I was miserable. The truth of Trina's accusation seemed to permeate my whole life, at camp and everywhere else. Every year I became more aware of my inability to fit in with the others who shared my camp sessions.

As I became more aware, the accusation became less true.

The year I was 16 I went to Spanish camp. It was the site at Cass Lake, where I had been before, and I knew the place and many of the counselors. Nothing had prepared me for the discovery I made there, of how much I had changed in my ability to interact.

It is puzzling that I have almost no memories of getting to know the other campers that year. Perhaps I slipped into this new life so perfectly, like a diver who enters the water without making a splash, that the beginning made no impact on my mind.

What I remember is how suddenly I was popular. It was as if I had spontaneously begun to radiate some pheromone that made me seem like the cleverest, nicest, most attractive person around. It astonished me. Suddenly, people wanted to talk with me, thinking everything I said was brilliant, and even tolerated my differences. One evening I had a serious outburst of hyperactivity and ran around the room for half an hour singing some nonsense song, and everyone just smiled and let it pass. That session, there was no one who saw me act weird and immediately rejected me. People actually cared about getting to know me as a person.

"Juanita" became a particularly close friend. Juanita wasn't her real name; everyone at Spanish camp got to have a Spanish pseudonym. She was short, skinny in a compact way, with short, curly dark brown hair and a slightly masculine but deeply sympathetic face. Above all, I remember her admiration for me, her conviction that I was infinitely kind and dazzlingly intelligent, and I remember that she showered me with compliments.

At the campfire one night, the group was singing a song containing the words "Qué guay!" which mean "How cool!" in the dialect of some parts of Spain. They sound, however, like the letters "KY," and, driven by a sudden impulse, I yelled out "Jelly!" If that had happened at an earlier session there might have been derisive giggles, embarrassed grimaces, reproaches from my cabinmates, reprimands from the staff, or all four. But this time Juanita, who was sitting next to me, burst into laughter, applauded me for my cleverness, and later related the story with delight to our cabinmates, without a trace of the ridicule there would have been a year earlier.

I remember an incredible sense of harmony and peace throughout the entire session. It was not an uneventful session—that was the year that my fainting spells became severe enough to arouse medical concern, and I had to go home for a couple days in the middle of the four-week session to see neurologists. But I remember everyone's deep concern for me and how I became homesick for camp during the days I was at home, while most years I spent a great deal of my time at camp being homesick for Minneapolis.

And there was Pablo.

Pablo was his Spanish pseudonym, not his real name, but it is how I have always thought of him. He was unusually tall; even his face was tall, with features somewhat too small for it, and curly, sand-brown hair.

We walked around together all the time, talking to each other in Spanish, even though most campers would lapse into English as soon as there were no counselors around. I can't remember the things we talked about. I don't even remember if I thought of him as anything more than a friend, until one day one of the little two-week campers saw us walking together and asked, "Hey, is that your girlfriend?"

Pablo and I looked at each other, and then he held my hand and said "Yes." And I do remember that it seemed like the perfectly natural thing for him to say.

A few days later, we were sitting at the picnic table under the big cedar tree by the central lodge, eating peach-flavored chewy candies. I found myself leaning close to him, and suddenly we found ourselves kissing, with open mouths, with our tongues. It didn't feel sudden, but seemed to flow smoothly from the previous moments in an almost relaxing way.

Afterwards I asked him, "Have you ever kissed anyone before?"

"No," he answered.

"Neither have I," I said.

It was true. And yet we were still so calm that we'd spoken in Spanish.

We kissed at every possible opportunity for the rest of the session. Without ever talking about it, we developed a code of body language: when I leaned my head against his neck, it meant I wanted him to kiss me, and he understood. We kissed in public, so addicted to the new feeling that we didn't care what other people thought. We kissed in the nurse's office when I was sick for a few days and he was allowed in to see me. We kissed once when I was wearing my retainer, and I didn't realize I was wearing it until his tongue was in my mouth. Then we stopped kissing and I took the retainer out and stood there confused, wondering whether to put it back in or kiss him again, and we laughed.

We lay down in the grass behind some little building at the Norwegian camp that we all went to for "International Day," and kissed until ants started biting me and I had to get up and jump around and shake them off me. We sat together on a bench, at the dance on the last night of the camp session, leaning on each other, embracing, every once in a while kissing until the counselors made us stop.

Then I went home to Minneapolis, and he went home to New Jersey. We tried to keep in touch through email, but I had no internet access of my own, and could only go online when Mom took me to her office. Infrequent as this made our correspondence, it got even less frequent as time went on, and finally stopped.

I kept in touch longer with Juanita; I wrote to her from every subsequent camp session, and we even sent each other gifts sometimes. But we, too, grew apart, long enough ago that I don't even remember her real name.

The feeling of being loved by everyone has remained in my memory, though. In the years since then, and the many groups of people I have associated with, I have not always been popular. Sometimes I have needed to get to know a new group of friends very well before they've accepted me to that degree. There have been bad social experiences, and there have been ones even better than that session at Spanish camp. But I will always remember it as the first time.

Friends

I remember the first time I slept over at a friend's house. I was in kindergarten. The friend, Elena, was a classmate. I remember her as dark and energetic, with a mass of curly black hair and a vivacious personality. I was five; she was probably six. My mother engineered the sleepover, desperate for me to have a friend.

It was Elena's birthday. The evening began at Chuck E Cheese's, a place my parents never took me, a place I had even been taught to dislike. Considering that my mother knew I was going there and didn't object, she must not have hated it too much, so I wasn't worried.

Elena and I rushed happily from room to room, catching glimpses of video-game machines, ball-throwing challenges, glass boxes full of stuffed animals that you could try to lift out with a mechanical arm. We had no money, but seeing things was enough fun!

Some friend or relative of hers gave me a coin, and I put it in a machine that contained a mechanical chicken on a pile of eggs. The chicken clucked and fluffed its feathers, and an egg rolled out for me; I opened it to find a plastic toy. I think it was a little red horse.

The next thing I remember we were at her house, playing in her room prior to going to bed. Her room looked like the girls' section of a toy shop. Everything was very pink, very feminine, very neatly organized. Dolls. Makeup sets. Books about ballerinas. We pretended to be in a jewelry store, and she showed me all her bright, sparkly plastic beads.

I was fascinated. She had so many more pretty things than I did. My parents may have bought me all the books and art supplies I wanted, but they had neglected me where pink plastic toys were concerned.

The only thing in her jewelry box that I recognized was a set of pop-beads; each had a tiny knob on one end and a tiny hole on the other, so that they could be popped together into a necklace. There was a set of those at my house too; perhaps my mom had them from her childhood.

Elena took one and held it up. "I'm going to pierce your ears now," she announced. "Do you know how ears get pierced?"

"You put earrings in them," I answered. At that age I thought that the holes in pierced ears came from the first pierced earrings one ever wore.

"But first you have to do this," Elena explained. "You make a hole with this."

"That's a pop-bead," I protested.

"It's a special kind," she said patiently. She pushed the knob of the pop-bead against one of my earlobes, then the other. "That didn't hurt, did it?"

Looking in the mirror, I said, "I don't see any holes."

"The holes are too small to see," she replied.

For months, I believed I had pierced ears.

Days later, we were at kindergarten, playing together by ourselves. "You have to learn to eat paper," she told me.

"How do you eat paper?"

"You just take a little bit of it, and rip it off, and put it in your mouth. Chew it up until it's nice and wet, and then swallow it. It's great."

When I ate paper in front of the other kids, they laughed at me.

"Elena told me to," I defended myself.

"I didn't mean really," cried Elena. "I was just pretending."

Part of my trouble relating to other children was that I didn't understand their ways of pretending. I pretended mostly alone, by telling myself made-up stories, or directing dramas in which the main characters were my toys (or even my hands, with their fingers opening and closing to look like the mouths of animals).

Sometimes I pretended with my brother, but our fantasies were outlandish enough never to be confused with reality. We never started pretending without announcing it: "Let's play that we're dinosaurs!" "Let's play that we're traveling to the bottom of the ocean!"

In any case, it was many years before I had a sleepover again, even though I did have a few friends in grade school—girls who were as weird as I was, or, more often, girls with such an abundance of social skills that they could look past my obvious differences and see the attractive traits I did possess.

These were the children who saw me as an individual, a person of my own, instead of some stereotype of abnormality. They listened to me, talked with me, truly got to know me. They admired me for my wild imagination, they found me fun to be with, and I was grateful to them for paying attention to me.

We seldom went to each other's houses. We had our fun making up secret codes and ciphers, passing notes to each other that nobody else could read. We drew pictures and wrote stories and showed them to each other. We made treasure chests: jars full of coins or toys or plastic jewels, and buried them in the sand on the playground. We tried to find them later; sometimes we succeeded, sometimes not.

Such friends were merciful exceptions to the rule that I fit in with nobody. I am grateful to them and always will be; without their friendship, my only enjoyable interaction would have been with close family members and a few teachers.

Yet I never stayed with these friends long. Often I came to school the next year to find that they were not in my class. Several times my parents found a different school and moved me there, hoping it would be better for me. In those cases I forgot the people I had played with in the old setting and formed whatever new friendships I could form where I was.

Only a few precious friends stayed with me longer. Lucy, whom I met in fourth or fifth grade, was the first of these.

Lucy's hair was long, brown, and always neatly combed; she wore lacy blouses and subtle jewelry like a tiny gold heart on a thin chain. She was, I believe, of British ancestry, and loved British twists of language.

"I sometimes put hyphens in words when I write," she admitted to me, "like 'pillow-case,' or 'doll-house.' I like the way it looks. It's so much prettier."

Another time I laughed about flushing something down the toilet, and she interrupted me. "The *loo*," she corrected, laughing with me. "Flush it down the loo."

She loved the work of the children's author Roald Dahl, and introduced me to many of his books, from *Witches* to *The Twits.* In contrast to Dahl's characters, she was one of the sweetest, most refined and gentle people I have ever known.

The very idea of associating pigs with her was hilarious, which may have been why she and I gave each other so many pig-related gifts over the years. Stuffed pigs, pig figurines, books about pigs, even pig jewelry.

I lost most of the things she gave me, but in a drawer I still have one of them: a flat piece of wood, painted red and cut into the outline of a pig. It was a brooch, although it has lost the pin on the back by now.

In high school English class, taught by the brilliant Mr. Froehle, I met two new friends. One was Christina: dark-haired, impeccably polite and friendly, and as ladylike as Lucy. She and I worked together on assignments, had lunch together sometimes, and invited each other to birthday gatherings. Sometimes Lucy joined us, and it was a regular British tea party.

The other friend, Ali, was someone completely different. I had gone to junior high school with her, but I'd hardly known her then. She was one of the smallest, thinnest women I've met, but not by choice; she ate several large meals a day and snacked almost constantly to satisfy her raging metabolism.

Ali's hair was never the same twice. "It was black when I was a baby," she said. "Then it turned blond, then red, then brown. All by itself." I saw it go through several more changes, guided this time by Ali: it was dyed black, it grew long, then it was cut almost to the scalp, then grew out a bit and became wildly frizzy. For a while it was short and curly and golden-brown, with reddish highlights from time to time. Then it grew very long for a few months, and finally ended up medium-length and similar in color to mine.

Ali wore lots of makeup and very tight clothes, but not to attract boys or to defy her parents. She had no interest in any young man who would notice her only because of her outfit. Her parents fully approved of her wearing whatever she liked. She dressed up purely for herself, because she liked the way she looked in those clothes. She was strong, outspoken, and argumentative, always ready to defend anything about her that came into question.

Ali was two years younger than I. Everyone assumed that I was a sort of mentor for her. Talking about Christina, Mr. Froehle said to me, "You two seem made for each other. I'm so glad you've become friends; you get along so well." Talking about Ali, he said, "Be a pal to Ali, okay? Help her understand things. She respects you a lot."

If I helped her, it was the help that anyone gets from having a good friend, the same help she gave to me. I didn't have to explain to Ali how the world worked; she could figure that out on her own just as well as I could. I wasn't any more of a sympathetic ear for her troubles than she was for mine. We were simply friends, and our friendship has lasted longer than any of the others. What brought us together was the realization that we both created worlds.

As I said earlier, I had invented several alien species: the Erilcans, the Andromedians, the Springers. I had written thick journals full of information about their cultures; painted and drawn pictures of them; made some of the things they made, like their clothing and jewelry. Ali, meanwhile, had invented the Xthions, the Valerians, and dozens of other species that she had immortalized in works of short fiction.

My cousins and I had pretended that my basement bedroom was "Shuttlecraft Investigator of the Galactica Starbase." We all had ranks and titles aboard it and alien species of our own. I was Captain Terri, an Andromedian. My cousin Matthew was First Officer Rombis, a Camelin. My cousin Sonja was a communications officer named Alicia who had hatched from a pod on a tree on Planet Zero. My cousin Carly—Doctor Linsla—was an Erilcan. My cousin Peter was Lieutenant-commander Retep, a Fire Lizard, born on a sun called Starbow 2. My cousin David, who called himself Engineer Ben, was the only human on the shuttle.

Independently of me, Ali and her family had done almost the same thing. She was an Xthion called First Officer Clia; her mother was an admiral and her father was a captain, without species specified. Her sister changed name, rank, and species frequently. Their imaginary spaceship had several other officers with no real people to represent them; they showed up only in the stories Ali wrote.

Once Ali and I became friends, one of our favorite activities was working on our imagined universes together. She told me scenarios from her universe, and I drew pictures of them for her. She colored the pictures and added details to suit herself.

Ali showed me stories she had written, and I wrote new ones to go with them. First, the stories I wrote involved only her characters, but later I brought our worlds together. In one story, her ship discovered a portal to an alternate universe, which turned out to be the universe in which my shuttle and its crew existed. From then on, they often visited each other in our writings.

Ali had been diagnosed with Asperger's Syndrome. Later she was given other tests, and her doctors decided on a different diagnosis that suited her better. I still think she has some Asperger's characteristics, but I don't know all the details, and I don't plan to argue with her. What's important is that she's doing well in her education, has a promising future, and is still one of my best friends in the world.

Ali ended up going to the same college I've been going to. There, through her, I've met Marie, my other kindred spirit. In some ways, she may be even more like me.

In all the time I have known Marie, her hair has stayed the same color and length: almost black, quite thick, reaching nearly to her shoulders. Marie is not as thin as Ali; she has a pleasant round face, and I never think of her without picturing bright eyes and a cheerful smile. She wears flowing, loose clothing with patterns and shapes that remind me just slightly of medieval times. When she wears jewelry, it often has some mystical symbolism: a five-pointed star, an ancient rune.

Where Ali fights and stands up for herself, Marie is calmer. Like me, she might remain silent while someone says something stupid or mean, and only later recount that unpleasant speech to her friends, so we can share in the ranting and ridiculing.

Marie clearly has Asperger's. Like me, she has learned to fit in to a certain degree, but little things about her are still "just a little off." She talks a little too loudly; laughs a little too much in places a laugh doesn't belong, and she sometimes continues talking long after people have lost interest. She also repeats some thoughts a few times. Marie is not quite sure when people are done talking or want to begin talking again, so she finds herself interrupting sometimes.

Marie and I share many of the little, almost unimportant remnants of disorders that once made a cage of both our lives. And we share some interests.

Marie likes science fiction and fantasy. Her main hobby is collecting names. Whenever she meets someone with a name she finds interesting or pleasant, she stores it in a list she keeps on her computer. She looks through name books and novels for new additions to her collection.

Marie and I don't usually write and draw together. My conversations with her are about many things: philosophy, politics, religion, love, sex, nature, art ... and of course the many quirks of Earthling society and our attempts to fit in.

I'm deeply grateful to have friends who have gone through some of the same difficulties I have, learning the foreign language of human life, teaching others the language of ourselves. My friends and I have come a long way, and with each other's help and the help of many other people, we've finally made Earth a place that can feel like home to us.

Becoming an Earthling

I have finally settled in on Earth, overcome my culture shock, and started making friends with these fascinating creatures called humans. My life has been a rigorous naturalization process in which I have gone from being an alien to becoming a citizen of this planet.

I used to be unable to carry on a normal conversation. I talked far too loudly, repeated the beginnings of phrases, didn't make the right noises and facial expressions in response to other people's words, bragged about myself, and got into unnecessary arguments.

Now I can talk just fine. When I have something interesting to say, which is often, my family and friends love to sit and listen to me, asking dozens of questions, hoping to draw my conversation out. I am still a bit loud, and my facial expressions and "Uh-huh" and "Mm-hmm" noises are not quite right, but people just get the impression that I am a bit eccentric. Nobody has ever called me a bad conversationalist.

I used to go into rages at the slightest annoyance. I hit and bit people, or struggled so hard not to hit or bite them that I ached all over. Tiny things brought me to a fever pitch of anger, like being teased about my clothes or being told by a teacher that spiders were insects.

Now I am an easygoing person. If someone yells at me or expresses an opinion that makes no sense to me I listen politely, then wait until I am alone with a friend to complain about it. It is quite rare for me to feel so angry that I hurt, and I never get so angry that I hurt other people.

I used to have no idea how to joke; I ended up threatening or insulting people by mistake. I had seen a cousin playfully pointing a fork at a sibling who had just snatched a piece of food off her plate, and saying "I'm gonna kill you for that." I tried shouting the same words while grasping a knife and leaping out from around a corner at someone. I couldn't understand why my cousin's joke was funny and mine wasn't.

Now I have a good understanding of jokes. My sense of humor is what my friends like most about me. I'm still sometimes not sure what is the best joke for a certain group or situation, but I have a wide repertoire of funny things to say: jokes I've invented, quotes from other people, even some comic poetry of my own. I can be the life of a party without getting drunk. I can be a class clown without getting a bad grade.

I used to go out of my way to look attractive and fail utterly: my clothes and makeup were way overdone and never matched. I looked like someone dressing up as a prostitute for a skit, and I thought I was just elegantly beautiful.

Now I can look very beautiful if I want to, and my friends shower me with compliments each time I try it. But usually I don't bother. I prefer hanging out in comfortable T-shirts and jeans. I would rather have people like me for my mind than for my clothes, and when I don't dress up I can be sure that's what's happening.

I have become a person who can function socially on this planet, sometimes with great success. There are times when I'm not sure what I should do; there are times when I am a bit awkward, but that happens to all humans, and I do quite well for somebody who didn't feel like a human at first.

I can't say if I feel like a human now. I have never been a normal human, and I don't know how it feels to be one. I feel like me. And I feel much more comfortable with humans than I used to. Even if I was meant to be on another planet, I have certainly made the best of living on this one.

I don't know if I was put on the wrong planet literally—if, through some cosmic mistake, a soul that belonged in another galaxy ended up being born to Dr. Mary Arneson and Dr. Dale Hammerschmidt of Minneapolis, Minnesota. I don't know if there truly is a planet somewhere out in space where I would fit in better. All I know is that I have taken many years to learn to fit in on the planet Earth.

When I think of myself as an alien, it is a way of putting a name to the struggles of those years. I can say that I was born without the instincts for human social interaction because my soul wasn't meant to interact with humans; it was meant to be born among creatures on some far-off world. I can say that I have attacks of hyperactivity because they are a regular occurrence among members of my true species, as routine as the monthly cycle of human females. I can say that my linguistic savant skills are alien powers, normal on my planet but above average on Earth.

I can say that it is possible for an alien to learn to fit in on Earth, just as it is possible for an Earthling to move from one country to another and learn to fit in there. It isn't easy, and the change will never be complete. Traces of the old patterns will remain in one's speech and behavior as long as one lives; traces of prejudice against foreigners will remain in the natives of one's new home.

The longer one stays in a foreign place, the more one becomes a part of that culture. I have become a part of this one, a part that's bright and colorful and stands out proudly, but that still connects firmly to the parts around her.

If you have Tourette's, Asperger's, ADD, ADHD, OCD, or any other trait that makes you feel alien, that doesn't negate your potential as a successful human being or your ability to realize that potential. It doesn't take away your ability to be happy—you just need confidence in yourself and the support of those who love you. There is effort involved, but it's worth it. Most of all, never feel that you have to be like everyone else. Uniqueness is one of your greatest treasures, and diversity is what makes the world truly enjoyable.

Appendix

What is Asperger Syndrome?

Asperger Syndrome (AS), also called Asperger's Disorder, is a neurobiological disorder named for a Viennese physician, Hans Asperger, who in 1944 published a paper that described a pattern of behaviors in several young boys who had normal intelligence and language development, but who also exhibited autistic-like behaviors and marked deficiencies in social and communication skills. In spite of the publication of his paper in the 1940s, it wasn't until 1994 that Asperger Syndrome was added to the DSM IV and only in the past few years has AS been recognized by professionals and parents.

Individuals with AS can exhibit a variety of characteristics and the disorder can range from mild to severe. Persons with AS show marked deficiencies in social skills, have difficulties with transitions or changes and prefer sameness. They often have obsessive routines and may be preoccupied with a particular subject of interest. They have a great deal of difficulty reading nonverbal cues (body language) and very often the individual with AS has difficulty determining proper body space. Often overly sensitive to sounds, tastes, smells, and sights, the person with AS may prefer soft clothing, certain foods, and be bothered by sounds or lights no one else seems to hear or see.

It's important to remember that the person with AS perceives the world very differently. Therefore, many behaviors that seem odd or unusual are due to those neurological differences and not the result of intentional rudeness or bad behavior, and most certainly not the result of "improper parenting."

By definition, those with AS have a normal IQ and many individuals (although not all), exhibit exceptional skill or talent in a specific area. Because of their high degree of functionality and their naiveté, those with AS are often viewed as eccentric or odd and can easily become victims of teasing and bullying. While language development seems, on the surface, normal, individuals with AS often have deficits in pragmatics and prosody. Vocabularies may be extraordinarily rich and some children sound like "little professors." However, persons with AS can be extremely literal and have difficulty using language in a social context. At this time there is a great deal of debate as to exactly where AS fits. It is presently described as an autism spectrum disorder and Uta Frith, in her book *Autism and Asperger's Syndrome*, described AS individuals as "having a dash of Autism." Some professionals feel that AS is the same as High Functioning Autism (HFA) while others feel that it is better described as a Nonverbal Learning Disability (NLD). AS shares many of the characteristics of PDD-NOS (Pervasive Developmental Disorder; Not Otherwise Specified), HFA, and NLD and because it was virtually unknown until a few years ago, many individuals either received an incorrect diagnosis or remained undiagnosed. For example, it is not at all uncommon for a child who was initially diagnosed with ADD or ADHD be rediagnosed with AS. In addition, some individuals who were originally diagnosed with HFA or PDD-NOS are now being given the AS diagnosis and many individuals have a dual diagnosis of Asperger Syndrome and High Functioning Autism.

Tourette's Syndrome

Tourette's Syndrome is an inherited, neurological disorder characterized by repeated and involuntary body movements (tics) and uncontrollable vocal sounds. In a minority of cases, the vocalizations can include socially inappropriate words and phrases, called coprolalia. These outbursts are neither intentional nor purposeful. Involuntary symptoms can include eye blinking, repeated throat clearing or sniffing, arm thrusting, kicking movements, shoulder shrugging, or jumping.

These and other symptoms typically appear before the age of 18 and the condition occurs in all ethnic groups with males affected three to four times more often than females. Although the symptoms of TS vary from person to person and range from very mild to severe, the majority of cases fall into the mild category. Associated conditions can include attentional problems, impulsiveness, and learning disabilities.

Most people with TS lead productive lives and participate in all professions. Increased public understanding and tolerance of TS symptoms are of paramount importance to people with Tourette's Syndrome.

Asperger's Disorder

Diagnostic Features

The essential features of Asperger's Disorder are severe and sustained impairment in social interaction (Criterion A) and the development of restricted, repetitive patterns of behavior, interests, and activities (Criterion B).... The disturbance must cause clinically significant impairment in social, occupational, or other important areas of functioning (Criterion C). In contrast to Autistic Disorder, there are no clinically significant delays in language (e.g., single words are used by age 2 years, communicative phrases are used by age 3 years) (Criterion D). In addition, there are no clinically significant delays in cognitive development or in the development of age-appropriate self-help skills, adaptive behavior (other than in social interaction), and curiosity about the environment in childhood (Criterion E). The diagnosis is not given if the criteria are met for any other specific Pervasive Developmental Disorder or for Schizophrenia (Criterion F).

Tourette's Disorder

Diagnostic Features

The essential features of Tourette's Disorder are multiple motor tics and one or more vocal tics (Criterion A). These may appear simultaneously or at different periods during the illness. The tics occur many times a day, recurrently throughout a period of more than one year (Criterion B). During this period, there is never a tic-free period of more than three consecutive months. The disturbance causes marked distress or significant impairment in social, occupational, or other important areas of functioning (Criterion C). The onset of the disorder is before age 18 years (Criterion D). The tics are not due to the direct physiological effects of a substance (e.g., stimulants) or a general medical condition (e.g., Huntington's disease or postviral encephalitis) (Criterion E).

The anatomical location, number, frequency, complexity, and severity of the tics change over time. The tics typically involve the head and, frequently, other parts of the body, such as the torso and upper and lower limbs. The vocal tics include various words or sounds such as clicks, grunts, yelps, barks, sniffs, snorts, and coughs. Coprolalia, a complex vocal tic involving the uttering of obscenities, is present in a few individuals (less than 10%) with this disorder. Complex motor tics involving touching, squatting, deep knee bends, retracing steps, and twirling when walking may be present. In approximately one-half of the individuals with this disorder, the first symptoms to appear are bouts of a single tic, most frequently eye blinking, less frequently tics involving another part of the face or the body. Initial symptoms can also include tongue protrusion, squatting, sniffing, hopping, skipping, throat clearing, stuttering, uttering sounds or words, and coprolalia. Other cases begin with multiple symptoms.

Obsessive-Compulsive Disorder

Diagnostic Features

The essential features of Obsessive-Compulsive Disorder are recurrent obsessions or compulsions (Criteria A) that are severe enough to be time consuming (i.e., they take more than 1 hour a day) or cause marked distress or significant impairment (Criterion C). At some point during the course of the disorder, the person has recognized that the obsessions or compulsions are excessive or unreasonable (Criterion B). If another Axis I disorder is present, the content of the obsessions or compulsions is not restricted to it (Criterion D). The disturbance is not due to the direct physiological effects of a substance (e.g., a drug of abuse, a medication) or a general medical condition (Criterion E).

Attention-Deficit/Hyperactivity Disorder

Diagnostic Features

The essential feature of Attention-Deficit/Hyperactivity Disorder is a persistent pattern of inattention and/or hyperactivity-impulsivity that is more frequent and severe than is typically observed in individuals at a comparable level of development (Criterion A). Some hyperactive-impulsive or inattentive symptoms that cause impairment must have been present before age 7 years, although many individuals are diagnosed after the symptoms have been present for a number of years (Criterion B). The disturbance does not occur exclusively during the course of a Pervasive Developmental Disorder, Schizophrenia, or other Psychotic Disorder and is not better accounted for by another mental disorder (e.g., a Mood Disorder, Anxiety Disorder, Dissociative Disorder, or Personality Disorder) (Criterion E).

Afterword

Being the parent of a child with ADD or ADHD, Asperger's or Tourettes, or the parent of an autistic child is, in spite of what everyone says parenthood is supposed to be, a frustrating and often maddening experience!

Likewise, I am told by my son, it is a frustrating and tension-producing experience being the sufferer. For much of your life, people think you're weird, and you can't figure out why, and you spend a lot of time being angry and even hitting out at things around you, which just makes things much worse. The way you see the world makes perfect sense to you, even if it is not the way you are supposed to see the world. And who says the world is that way anyway?

An unconventional perspective is not something that gets you through school easily, as Erika Hammerschmidt points out. Nor does it get you through day-to-day relationships, or help you make friends.

On either side of this equation, you spend most of your time worrying. If you are the parent, you worry about what will become of your child. If you are the sufferer, you worry about what will become of you. Unfortunately, professional advice often seems empty and irrelevant!

When I first read this book, I started laughing. For the first time in a long time, I began to see a light at the end of a very dark tunnel.

In this short book, Erika Hammerschmidt describes what can and *will* happen, if there is a very great effort from both family and afflicted. And the news is good!

Erika Hammerschmidt writes from the inside — not as a professional, but as someone with a whole host of problems. She writes as a young woman who, at 21, in spite of her collection of symptoms and problems, submitted a 300-page book and completely and cheerfully revamped it in just a few months (a daunting task for any author). Erika Hammerschmidt speaks several languages, and studies in Germany, Spain, and, I imagine, pretty much anywhere else she wants to go. She looks at the world through the eyes of someone with a handicap using resources to do what she wants to do in life even though her brain is wired a little strangely.

The most valuable thing I gained from this book is perspective. I began to relax. I started dealing with my son a little differently. When I am thoroughly frustrated with something he does, I hear Erika Hammerschmidt's voice in the back of my mind. When I am ready to yell, "Don't you know what you did wrong?" there is Erika Hammerschmidt's voice saying "No. He doesn't. Be a little patient. He will."

That there are a lot of very creative scientists and artists who have ADD or Asperger's, or even problems with being bipolar, is not something that particularly helps me deal with the day-to-day frustrations of worrying about my son. But after reading Erika Hammerschmidt's book, it occurs to me that those whom the gods wish to honor (to take the classic phrase just a little out of context), they first make strange!

What of the title? I almost asked the author to change it, but as an afterthought one afternoon, I handed the manuscript to my son Michael, and asked him to read it and let me know what he thought from his own view on the inside. A few hours later, he brought it back.

"Don't change the title," he said.

"Why not?"

"Because it's how a lot of people feel, me included!"

And so here you have "Born on the Wrong Planet," which is one young woman's journey through the first part of a pretty successful life, little by little, with a handicap that beats a lot of people. I hope you enjoy this book as much as I have, and that it makes you feel, if you do not feel that way already, that these disorders need not paralyze anyone, or keep them from achieving their full potential as individuals, a potential that is, possibly, quite a bit higher than that of some so-called normal people!

Raphael E. Serebreny
Publisher
Tyborne Hill Publishers
Palo Alto, California
March 2005

More from Erika Hammerschmidt

INSIDE

A CD Audio view of life from Erika Hammerschmidt's personal perspective!

If you enjoyed *Born on the Wrong Planet,* you will enjoy hearing Erika Hammerschmidt. Her new CD Audio **Inside** is available from Tyborne Hill.

Inside is a 45 minute presentation given in November of 2004 in front of an audience of 200 people in California. Sitting alone at a table, Erika Hammerschmidt charmed her entire audience:

"She told her story in a way that brought both laughter and tears. She has a passion for her subject that only one who has lived her life could express. Edie Bader, MA

Available for $11.00 plus shipping and handling, **Inside**, is a perfect companion for *Born on the Wrong Planet.*

Order online from www.tybornehill.com or send a check for $11.00 plus $4.00 shipping and handling to:

Tyborne Hill Publishers
2730 South Court Street
Palo Alto, California 94306

California residents add 8.25% sales tax. No credit cards on direct orders; personal checks welcome. Credit cards accepted online, price of CD is slightly higher.